Public Privates

Public Privates

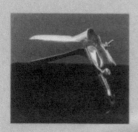

PERFORMING GYNECOLOGY

DUKE UNIVERSITY PRESS   Durham and London 1997

FROM BOTH ENDS OF THE SPECULUM

by Terri Kapsalis

© 1997 Duke University Press
All rights reserved
Printed in the United States of America on acid-free paper ∞
Typeset in Minion by Wilsted & Taylor
Frontispiece photo by Glenda Kapsalis
Library of Congress Cataloging-in-Publication Data appear
on the last printed page of this book.

For
Alvina Sophie Libert Hawley
and
Eleftheria Bravakou Kapsali

Contents

Acknowledgments

As a member of Theater Oobleck, an experimental theater collective, I learned how to make theater without a director. Collective members and their friends would sit in on rehearsals, serving as "outside eyes." Outside eyes would offer their opinions and input throughout the process of putting together a play. But "actor's prerogative" prevailed, meaning that the performer would incorporate those notes she felt helpful but, in the end, she was the one responsible to what she had created. It is in this spirit that this book was written. Its production would not have been possible without these outside eyes:

Margaret Drewal (for phenomenal support and potlucks), Dwight Conquergood (for continual encouragement), Lisa Cartwright (THANK YOU), Lillian Lennox (for vulvamorphic excursions), Mary Lass Stewart, Pam Robertson, Gretchen Long, Anna McCarthy, Karen Andes, Leslie Ashbaugh, Holly Clayson, Mimi White, Chrissie Richards, Ora Schub, Brenda Darrell, Louise Champlin, Sharon Powell, Joan Nelson, Sandy McNabb, Judy Sculley, Laura McAlpine, Tanya McHale, Anne Eckman, Elizabeth Young, Cecelia Lawless, Chuck Kleinhans, Andrew Parker, David Grubbs, Gregory Whitehead, Mick and Katherine Hurbis-Cherrier, Kathleen Pirrie Adams, Annie Sprinkle, Pam Gilchrist, Chris Slawinski, and Sa Schloff.

For being so kind and for dusting the plaster from my forehead, many thanks:

Kevin Whitehead (for imprudent title suggestions), Dawn and Lou Mallozzi (for sonic relief), Sarah VonFremd (for tea relief), Robin Rosenblate (for a lifetime of desserts), Wylie Goodman (for sharing a treehouse), Rick Wojcik, Hal Rammel, Gina Litherland, Jaxson, Tnoona, Jake, Catherine Roberts, Tria Smith, Ken Vandermark, Ellen Major, Bruno Johnson, David Isaacson, Dave Buchen, Danny Thompson, Lisa Black, and all Ooblecks past and present.

Many thanks to my open and supportive family network: Effie Kapsalis, Glenda Kapsalis, Andreas Kapsalis, Jayne Hyland, Michael Fesi, Tim Fitzgerald, Mary Ellen Blanchard, Arlene Reinwald, Howard Reinwald, Kari Rosenblate, Howard Rosenblate, Lisa Bershe, Curt Bershe, Adam Hunter, James Corbett, Joyce Corbett, Jillian Corbett, and Jennifer Corbett.

Thanks to Ken Wissoker, Richard Morrison, the folks at Duke University Press, and the two anonymous readers who provided valuable comments.

Hats off to the wonderful women of the Northwestern Alumnae Foundation for having faith in this project and awarding me a much-needed dissertation grant. I am also grateful to have received a Northwestern dissertation year travel grant, which allowed me to visit such places as the Kinsey Institute.

Finally, endless thanks to my ever-prescient reader, editor, transfuser, and all around "big dig," John Corbett.

Public Privates

Introduction: Public Privates

Spend a week telling people you know and meet that you are working on a book about pelvic exams. If your experience is anything like mine, your statement will be met with a variety of reactions: nervous laughter, surprise, horror, blank stares, suggestive winks, embarrassment, anger, excitement, disgust, discomfort, absolute silence. But silence is rare, at least from women. Much more often stories come forth. Women I've just met will often offer me going-to-the-gynecologist tales. There are many genres of these stories: first pelvic exam "rite of passage" stories, inappropriate practitioner stories, pain stories, inept practitioner stories, wonderful practitioner stories, funny things that happened at the gynecologist stories, fear stories, and so on. These stories could comprise a book in and of themselves.

One story keeps coming back to me. She was at the gynecologist's, in position for an exam. Her heels were in footrests, knees open, drape sheet covering her legs, lying so that she could not see beyond her draped knees. In the middle of the exam, her physician was called away. Leaving her in this prone position with the drape raised, he told her he'd be right back. As he left, he did not close the exam room door all the way. The room was set up in such a way that anybody who walked down the office hallway would be able to see her exposed vulva. There was no apparent reason she had to stay in that position, no speculum was in place, no treatment was interrupted, but the doctor had not told her she could sit up or move so she did not. She thought there must have been a reason he left her in such a position. Her face became hot with embarrassment; she closed her eyes as she heard people walk back and forth outside the room. Eventually he came back, shut the door, and continued the exam. She did not say a word.

Like many stories about pelvic exams, this is a story about power and gender. As with many pelvic exam tales, this is a story about proper female performance. However, in this particular story, there is an implicit conundrum concerning how this woman should perform. To begin with, she resides in the position of spectacle. As Mary Russo notes, "Making a spectacle out of oneself seem[s] a specifically feminine danger. The danger [is] of an exposure."[1] In the pelvic exam the "exposure" is of the most troublesome and dangerous variety. The shame associated with an exposed vulva, or the mere suggestion of displaying that very priv̲━━━━━━━━━━ng. In a society that encourages women and little girls to k░░░░░░░░░er so that they are "good girls," only certain "kinds" of w░░░░░░░░kers and artists' models—willingly expose themselves in░░░░░

Traditionally, ░░ ░░░ ░░░░░text, proper female performance demands that a woman patient be compliant, that she do only what she is told to do. Part of that compliance within the pelvic exam entails the exposure of private parts—and the clinician has the power to make such demands. In this story, he has not granted the woman the right to sit up, remove her heels from the footrests, and place her legs together in order to prevent exposure. In this story, while torn about her choice, the woman decides that the execution of a compliant medical performance overshadows the risk of an exposed vulva. Or perhaps, putting the fact of her feelings of embarrassment and humiliation aside, her performance could be read very differently. Sustaining her vulnerable position could be seen as a resistant performance, an act of defiance. In other words, she enlists an image of proper medical performance in order to challenge notions of shameful public exposure of female privates. However, given the woman's feelings of embarrassment and anger, it is clear that the performance is not one of resistance or defiance; her silence about those feelings while at the physician's office completes her compliant performance.

This story locates the edge between the transgressive act of exposure and the submissive act of resignation. It reminds us that while multiple readings of every performance are possible, there are risks in ascribing too much resistance to what may be more aptly interpreted as an act of submission. And conversely, there are risks in ascribing too much compliance to what may be more fully understood as an act of dissent. The term "performance" highlights the idea that gynecological practice is constructed and open to multiple readings and inter-pretations. Far from static or given, gynecology is continuously negotiated by performers who are simultaneously agents actively making choices and subjects directed by institutional and other cultural forces. Performance is neither "not real" nor implicitly staged. As will become clear over the course of this work, performance refers to that continuum of everyday life practices and staged rep-resentations that constitute gynecology.

The public performance of female privates is a particularly troublesome act. Shame of exposure is written into the history of the very word used to describe female private parts. The term "pudendum," which is still used interchangeably with "female genitalia" and "vulva," is from the Latin *pudere* and literally means "that of which one ought to be ashamed." However, in the Oxford English Dic-tionary, the connection between the word "pubes," "in the sense 'adult men,' 'male population,'" and the word "publicus," relating to "public" and "popu-lus," is made. Thus "pubes," referring to the pubic area, signifies adult *male* par-ticipation in the public sphere. Whereas female pudenda are allegedly parts to be ashamed of and therefore kept private, male pubes represent a public presence. The etymological underpinnings of the words "pubes" and "pudendum" point to the differing ideas surrounding male and female genital display.

These etymologies point to the inherent problem of the female pelvic exam: It is a practice that *necessitates* the *public* exposure of the shameful female *pri-vates*. In this book, public exposure takes many forms. The public is composed of medical students and licensed clinicians, performance art goers and lay prac-titioners, cinematic spectators and self-helpers. The privates belong to any number of "patients," including slave women, trained educators, prostitutes, ca-davers, plastic dolls, actresses, anesthetized women, and artists. The variety found in these two lists of publics and privates reveals that gynecology has a higher profile than may be imagined. A frequent player in popular culture, gynecology is featured in numerous venues, including film and television, jokes, cartoons, pornography, news media, and staged performance. Gynecology is a charged object of popular cultural curiosity in which humor, fear, horror, and titillation all meet. Even when gynecology occurs in the not-as-public space of the exam room, its power is far-reaching; women have long been subject to its ideological effects through their examinations.

As we shall see, the boundaries between the outside and inside of the medical establishment are porous. Actual gynecological practice can influence popular representations of gynecology, as is the case with David Cronenberg's film *Dead Ringers*, based on the story of actual twin male gynecologists (see chapter 6). Likewise, popular representation, including pornography, can influence gynecological practice, as exemplified by the photographs that medical textbook editors solicited from porn star and performance artist Annie Sprinkle (see chapter 4). Practices from outside the bounds of medicine influence gynecology: in the 1970s prostitutes were hired to help teach medical students how to give pelvic exams (see chapter 3). Similarly, innovations arising from within traditional medicine are used outside medical practice: while the speculum, invented in the United States by James Marion Sims, the Father of Gynecology, allowed Sims to surgically experiment on unanesthetized slave women in his backyard hospital in Montgomery, Alabama, between 1845 and 1849 (see chapter 2), this very instrument was, in turn, adopted by women's health activists beginning in the 1960s as a tool for female self-help groups (see chapter 7) and used by Annie Sprinkle in her "Public Cervix Announcement" (see chapter 5). Thus the pelvic exam is not simply owned and operated by the medical establishment. Rather it has a currency outside the medical institution, allowing it to both influence and be shaped by a variety of other spheres, including art, pornography, prostitution, and woman-centered activism.

Why write a critical investigation of gynecology? Because gynecology is the quintessential examination of women. Gynecology is not simply the study of women's bodies—gynecology *makes* female bodies. It defines and constitutes ▮▮▮▮▮▮▮▮▮▮ s critical examination of gynecology is simultaneously a ▮▮▮▮▮▮▮▮▮▮ t means to be female. Embedded in the varied perfor- ▮▮▮▮▮▮▮▮▮▮ re definitions of proper female performance. For each ▮▮▮▮▮▮▮▮▮▮ nce, a model patient is implied. In most contemporary circumstances in the United States, this ideal patient is insured, white, educated, mentally and physically able, thin, and heterosexual. In experimental situations, the model is often poor and a woman of color. Sims's surgical experiments are paradigmatic of this tendency; the institution of slavery provided the model women to whom Sims had unlimited surgical access.

In most cases the ideal patient is one who is compliant, passive, and accepting rather than active and questioning, a composite of proper womanly performance. This is perhaps epitomized in some of the "model patients" chosen by contemporary medical educators to teach students pelvic exams—cadavers, plastic dolls, and anesthetized women—models without feeling or feelings, models who can neither speak up nor act out. Whereas traditional pelvic exams are structured to both produce and reflect proper performances of womanliness, in a woman-centered alternative clinic model and in Annie Sprinkle's "Public Cervix Announcement" notions of the proper performance of the model female patient shift. In gynecology's many and varied practices and representations are found condensations of cultural attitudes and anxieties about women, female bodies, and female sexualities.

how
we view
adolescents
found in
sex ed.

As will be evident through an investigation of Sims's early practices, gynecology is traditionally a discipline concerned with mastering the female body. Such institutionalized power is intimately tied to making the mysteries of the female body visible and therefore knowable. Thus the "discovery" of the speculum allowed for the foundation of gynecology as a distinct specialty. Visibility leads to mastery. While Western medicine as a whole and the "birth of the clinic" are founded on visibility, as noted by Michel Foucault,[2] gynecology has a unique relationship to the art of making visible. The politics of gynecology and of making privates public is intimately related to the politics of vision and visibility. A critical investigation of gynecology—more specifically, pelvic exams—entails a consideration of what it means to expose what is normally hidden. *Public Privates* is about looking and being looked at, about speculums, spectacles, and spectators, about display, illumination, and reflection.

Built into the very materiality of the female body are contradictory themes related to visibility, themes that will appear throughout this work. The binary of lack and excess brings psychoanalytic claims about castration and absent penises in conversation with the excessive accoutrements of the pelvic realm: cervixes, secretions, folds, and vagina dentata. The paradox of inside and outside joins the asserted importance of making the vagina visible for medical exploration, experimentation, and intervention with cultural entrance taboos and fears of margins. Such contradictions surface throughout this text, highlighting the ways in which seemingly contradictory cultural constructions of femaleness constitute female anatomy.

The politics of visibility are variously inflected, shifting throughout the chapters of *Public Privates*. Fixed values cannot be attached to visibility. It is neither inherently good nor evil. The postmortem museum display of the dissected genitals of Saartje Baartman, popularly known as the Hottentot Venus, functions differently with regard to the politics of visibility than the spectacle of Annie Sprinkle's genitalia in the context of her performance art pieces. Making spectacles is about power, about who has the power to render visible and who has the power to look. Visibility can be oppression or liberation or both or neither. However, *Public Privates* is also about invisibility—about covering and masking, about anonymity and erasure. It is about being rendered invisible while residing in positions of glaring visibility. And this is also a book that recognizes the potential power of invisibility.[3]

And yet, *Public Privates* asserts the importance of making gynecology—its practices and representations—critically visible. Gynecology must be extracted from its private cover within clinic and hospital walls and medical textbook and history book pages into a broad public space of analysis and critique. Occasionally, when presenting portions of this work, I have encountered individuals who question the legitimacy of a nonmedical professional writing about gynecology. Too often gynecology is treated in this way: as something sacred to the medical establishment and therefore subject only to an internal gaze. This book suggests the necessity of critically addressing and redressing an institution to which so many of us are subject, of critically observing the numerous practices and representations that make gynecology, even if they are found behind closed doors, or behind doors that are meant to be closed.

I approach this topic not only as a medical consumer, but as an educator and performance practitioner. The idea for the project came to me in 1990 on the examination table. I was working as a gynecology teaching associate for a Chicago medical school, teaching a small group of second-year medical students breast and pelvic exam methods on my own body. The drape-sheet curtain was raised, the exam spotlight focused into the open speculum, the student-spectators were vying for a good view of my cervix, and, like a soundtrack, my voice was guiding them through the exercise. Amidst it all, I thought to myself, "What a performance." This performance was for me, at that time, one of political activism with distinct pedagogical and ideological aims, though now and then it felt more like a three-ring circus. Having recently begun graduate work at that time in performance studies, the connection was made between these two parts of my life, and the idea for this book materialized. Soon thereafter I became a member of a women's health collective, working as a health educator, teaching women breast and cervical self-exam. Through my experiences as a collective member at the clinic, my understanding of the politics of women's health has continued to shift and grow. All the while I have continued my work as a member of a Chicago-based experimental theater collective that still manages to complicate my understanding of the politics of staged performance and of what it means to make theater without a director. The sum of these experiences has contributed to this text, allowing for an invigorating exchange between its writing and these other performative modes.

In a 1978 article in the *American Journal of Obstetrics and Gynecology* a physician questions the role of the gynecology teaching associate, the role I was playing when the idea for this book struck: "My first question, as I suspect yours may be, was 'What *kind* of woman lets four or five novice medical students examine her?'" Perhaps the same question transformed will entertain the readers of this work: What *kind* of woman writes a book about pelvic exams? This is one of the project's many risks. Because of the charged nature of the topic, the writer risks association with the unseemly roles of voyeur and exhibitionist, of complicitous accomplice and resistant adversary. While the experience of writing this book

What kind of school does this?

has been one of both pleasure and horror, throughout the process the importance of critique has overridden whatever fear of images or dismay with certain
practices I might have felt. And there are reasons for writing about such a precarious topic, reasons that have spurred on this critical investigation of pelvic
exams.

Historically, gynecologists (along with psychiatrists, anatomists, etc.) have been
part of the group of experts who have constructed truths about women and their
bodies and sexualities. These experts are products of culture as well as cultural
producers. In part, therefore, gynecology is both a symptom of cultural attitudes
about women and their bodies as well as a means of perpetuating such attitudes.

Women have been and continue to be subject to gynecology. Gynecology, specifically the pelvic exam, helps construct women's experiences of their bodies
and sexualities. In addition, gynecology is the practice of treating women. How
women are perceived in turn directly affects their treatment.

Gynecological practices are repetitive and structured to situate the clinician and
object of the exam in very specific ways. In this sense, gynecology is a repeatable
performance with specific roles, scripts, sets, costumes, and props (see chapter
1). Although, depending on how they are perceived, women do receive differential treatment, specific aspects of medical practice are systematic and recurrent.
However, this idea that there are ways in which gynecology is a repeatable performance should not be held as evidence against the following reason.

Gynecology is not a singular or static entity and may be represented and prac-
ticed in a multiplicity of ways. This final reason is perhaps the one that most re-
wards the risks of writing about pelvic exams and gynecology. Because gynecology makes female bodies through its ubiquitous representations and practices,
it is one arena in which change may happen. Every time a pelvic exam occurs, be
it in a clinic, teaching hospital, small theater, or on a cinematic screen or textbook page, the potential exists to remake the pelvic exam performance and
therefore to reconfigure notions around proper female performance. Therefore
not only physicians but also performance artists, film directors, health activists,
midwives, nurse practitioners, patients, textbook editors, and pornographers
are cultural producers who make and remake gynecology. In so doing, they configure female bodies and sexualities. This critical investigation of gynecology and
a variety of its historical and contemporary medical and popular cultural practices and representations considers how female bodies and sexualities are made
and how they might be remade differently. However, this consideration of gynecology recognizes the tensions between individual performer's agency and repetitive structures, tensions that continually mediate the possibilities of change.
The final chapter is an exploration of some alternatives to traditional gynecol-

ogy. Rather than a prescription or panacea, this last chapter provides some possible and productive subversions of gynecological norms.

A number of related topics are touched upon throughout this work but are beyond the scope of the project. *Public Privates* invites a complementary exploration of the performances surrounding male genital examination and the constructions of male performance, bodies, and sexualities. Also, a consideration of the different modes of pedagogy and practice engaged in by nonphysician professionals such as nurse practitioners, midwives, and physician's assistants would add to what has been started here. While gynecology in the United States has had far-reaching international effects, *Public Privates* calls for explorations of gynecological practices and representations in other cultural and social contexts. Like gynecology, obstetrics is another powerful institution to which women have been subject, though I find it peculiar that much more critical work has been done on obstetric practice and representation than on gynecology. Obstetrics is largely beyond the scope of this book, but it lurks in the wings, relating and resounding in productive ways.

Public Privates is neither a comprehensive nor a complete examination of gynecology. Rather the various chapters form their own ensemble, performing a number of possible configurations of the pelvic exam. Many parallel books could be written; any number of ensembles are possible. My hope is that the unique ensemble formed in the following chapters will foster alternative performances and new possibilities.

1 The Performance of Pelvics

Dramaturgical Desexualization

In their 1971 article "Dramaturgical Desexualization: The Sociology of the Vaginal Examination," James M. Henslin and Mae A. Biggs considered the pelvic exam in theatrical terms, drawing on the work of Erving Goffman, an early performance theorist. They enlisted a dramaturgical model in order to focus on proper female patient performance and acceptable stagings of pelvic exams. Recognizing the dilemma of public privates, they concentrated on the "problematics of genital exposure" for the woman patient who must "expose her vagina in a nonsexual manner to a male."[1] Within the structure of the visit they found that a "dramaturgical desexualization" occurred in phases they labeled "scenes." While they divided the time the woman enters the waiting room until she leaves into nine steps, they maintained an overarching thematic: In order to desexualize the exam the woman must be transformed from "person to pelvic." After the exam, she may be transformed back into "person": "the individual is transformed from a full person into an object, into a 'person-possessing-a-pelvis' and even into a 'pelvis-that-incidentally-belongs-to-a-person.'"[2] Henslin and Biggs stress the importance of the drape sheet that covers the woman as a prop: "The drape sheet effectively hides [the patient's] pubic area *from herself* while exposing it to the doctor. With this, we have a beautiful example of a mechanism that effectively covers the pubic area for one actor while exposing it to the second."[3] Henslin and Biggs assert throughout the article that the patient must become separate from her pelvic region. In order to have a successful exam, as defined by Henslin and Biggs, the patient must become "a vagina disassociated from a person." The importance of careful and proper staging as well as meticulous role-playing and character shifting is emphasized repeatedly.

These authors do not critique pelvic exam dramaturgy. Rather they believe they are offering a truthful model of the ideal exam. Thus a "case of role failure" occurs when "the patient does not cooperate and play the role of object."[4] The example they use is that of a patient who has just undergone a surgical procedure to enlarge the vaginal opening, known as a hymenotomy. The patient in this case is a woman who is soon to be married and has had the surgery to make her first act of intercourse "easier." The patient is very upset and is exhibiting "uncooperative behavior" while the physician is attempting to examine her. The patient, her mother, the physician, and the nurse are all present during the exam. Apparently, Biggs herself served as a nurse during this exam as she did throughout the twelve thousand to fourteen thousand exams that Henslin and Biggs used as data. It is unclear whether this exam was documented (e.g., by sound recording) or whether Biggs transcribed the exam from memory. Nevertheless, the "case," appropriately formatted as a play script, reads as follows:

> The doctor enters the room and says, "When is that wedding going to be?" He pulls on his glove.
> The patient turns her head to the wall and mumbles, "The fifth of February."
> Doctor: "You should be completely healed by then." As the doctor starts to approach the patient, she moves back on the table away from him.
> Nurse: "Gerry, please bring your hips down."
> Doctor: "Come on, Gerry, bring your hips down."
> Patient: "I can't. It'll hurt."
> Doctor: "I'll be as careful as possible." The patient moves her hips down to the edge of the table. She closes her eyes tightly and tightly grips the edges of the table. The doctor inserts his fingers and begins the examination.
> Doctor: "Relax, Gerry, relax."
> Mother: "Come on, Gerry, he can't examine you if you act that way." The patient begins moving her head from side to side. The doctor starts to insert the speculum. The patient again moves her hips away from the doctor.
> Patient: "I can't! I can't!"
> Doctor: "Please relax so I can insert this speculum."

Mother: "Gerry! Quit acting like that!"

The patient again moves her hips to the edge of the table. The doctor carefully and slowly inserts the speculum.

Patient: "My God! You're tearing me apart! Give me something to bite on! Mom! Give me some gum!" (Patient is shaking her head from side to side very rapidly.) The mother reaches into her purse, removes some chewing gum, unwraps a piece and places it in the patient's mouth. The patient rapidly chews the gum. The nurse moves up to the abdominal area of the patient.

Nurse: "Gerry, please try to relax. It will be so much easier for you." The patient places her right arm over her eyes. Then she reaches out and grabs the nurse, digging her fingernails into the nurse's arm.

Patient: "He's ruining me! I can't stand it!" She continues to shake her head from side to side.

Doctor: "Gerry, I'm just trying to help you. This will be very helpful to you after you get married."

Patient: "I don't see how. It hurts too much."

Mother: "I'm sorry, doctor."

Doctor to Mother: "She's in good condition now. She'll take a normal sized speculum without difficulty." He withdraws the speculum and removes his glove. "I don't think I'll have to see her again—that is, unless she has difficulties later on."

Doctor to Patient: "Okay, Gerry, get dressed." The doctor touches her on her shoulder and says, "I want to have a long talk with you about your wedding." The patient closes her eyes and brings her arm over her eyes. The doctor then leaves the room.

The authors of the article then comment, "Fortunately for the success of the interaction flow such a refusal to accept the role of object—to be unresponding and uncomplaining—is rare. Almost always the projected definition of dramaturgical depersonalization is not only offered by the involved medical personnel but is also both eagerly accepted and cooperatively role-played by the patient."[5] The assertion throughout this article is that the only way a woman may be treated nonsexually is if she is desexualized by assuming the role of "unresponding and uncomplaining" object. Her sexualization is conflated with any activity that might steal her from the role of passive recipient of the exam. According to Henslin and Biggs, any exhibition of will or response whatsoever during the exam will inevitably undermine her desexualization, thus compromising her clinician. Ironically, however, the very procedure that Gerry has

undergone is medical preparation to ensure her ability to be properly penetrated by her husband and therefore enabling her sexual role as wife. If the script
were to continue and we were to follow a clothed Gerry into the physician's office
we would most likely find that his "long talk" with Gerry about her wedding
consisted of instructing Gerry as to her upcoming duties as wife and explaining
to her that the kind of behavior she exhibited during the exam would be unacceptable for the bridal bed. In other words, just as Henslin and Biggs criticized
Gerry for her failure to assume the role of unresponding and uncomplaining
object in the pelvic exam scenario, similarly this young bride-to-be will fail her
role of wife if she does not willingly submit to her husband's sexual demands. Be
it medical or heterosexual penetration, female role-failure is the risk. Gerry's behavior has been inappropriate in its execution of what Judith Butler refers to as
"the compulsory performance of woman." The compulsory performance of
woman, in Gerry's case, requires both mandatory heterosexuality and mandatory gynecology, events that must be accepted and endured without complaint.[6]

What becomes clear through a consideration of Gerry's case and Henslin and
Biggs's presentation of Gerry's case is that *the pelvic exam is in effect the staging of
sex and gender*, particularly the staging of femininity and female sexuality. Gerry's improper performance in the pelvic exam is simultaneously an improper
performance of womanliness. In addition, if the exam is not properly staged, if
Gerry or any other woman patient is not properly made into an object as Henslin and Biggs propose, the impropriety of the exam threatens the stability of its
medicalization. The public display of female privates is so troublesome that the
female patient must be properly rendered as an object or she poses a threat. Such
is the importance for Henslin and Biggs of locating those components of the pelvic exam's staging that they believe help medical personnel systematically "desexualize" the female patient, even (perhaps especially) when the surgery that
has been performed is expressly a move toward her hetero-sexualization.

The attempt to make Gerry into an uncomplaining and unresponding object
is in effect an attempt to make her into a prop for the physician's performance.
If proper staging occurred, as defined by Henslin and Biggs, Gerry would be
more like a prop for the physician's performance than a co-performer. Or if we
consider Gerry, costumed in her patient robe, to be a performer rather than a
prop, then the physician might be more appropriately cast as the director. He
oversees the exam, "blocks" the exam by arranging the various players, and
makes sure that they perform their roles properly. Considering the physician-as-
director acknowledges the differing power that the physician has in the exam
scenario. He is the one who, in most cases, runs the show. The physician's position of power within the exam is mirrored in the staging of the exam itself. The

set, consisting of exam table, stool, and so on, organizes the participants in disparate power-inflected positions. The physician sits on a stool while Gerry lies in lithotomy position: on her back with her heels in footrests, legs open.[7]

At times throughout the visit, the physician's role shifts to that of critic. Following the exam he will note pathologies in Gerry's chart. But even during the exam, he critiques Gerry's vaginal opening by stating that it may hold a normal size speculum and criticizes Gerry's behavior by suggesting they have a long talk about her wedding. In the case of physician-as-critic, the walls of the pelvic theater exceed the exam room walls, the clinic, and the hospital, extending into a variety of other institutions including the home, the state, and marriage.

Similarly the roles of Gerry's mother and the nurse are not static. In addition to their roles as co-performers, they join the physician as audience members and even critics. With this threesome as audience, the pelvic theater then largely occurs between Gerry's legs, which serve as wings of the pelvic proscenium. The drape-sheet curtain rises at the hands of the physician, dividing front stage from backstage, while the exam spotlight shines on the spectacle. The physician-spectator inserts a *spec*ulum and props open a little makeshift stage within a stage. In this space, a parallel drama occurs. Here is where the surgery has been performed, where instruments are plied, where little brushes and swabs sometimes dance like puppets at the hands of the physician. It is also where the drama of the wedding night will occur, the site of the defining performance of Gerry's heterosexualization.

The ideal patient then, according to Henslin and Biggs, would allow this proper pelvic theater to occur by keeping her eyes and voice and thoughts "backstage" to the exam in order to assume the position of passive object. However, Gerry's stage fright, which manifests itself in "inappropriate" behavior, disrupts a proper staging of this pelvic performance, complicating the physician's roles as director, critic, and audience member and forcing the mother and nurse to become more active participants and critics while spectating. Gerry herself is spectator to a different performance as she watches the drama unfold in the exam room. While completely disregarded by Henslin and Biggs, the significance of Gerry's role as spectator is not to be overlooked and will be investigated further in this chapter.

Henslin and Biggs limit all of the participants in Gerry's pelvic theater to the roles of co-performers or actors. However, they implicitly adopt hierarchies and power structures endemic to both traditional gynecology and traditional Western theater. Just as Henslin and Biggs have naturalized power relationships in the pelvic theater, so have they overlooked such relationships in the theater they use as metaphor for the vaginal exam. If we alter their metaphorical use of theater to

acknowledge the fact that roles shift throughout the exam—roles that, by definition, hold differing degrees of power—this allows for a more nuanced understanding of the pelvic production. Expanding the consideration of Gerry's case
to include positions such as director, critic, spectator, and prop provides for a
further comparison between the conventions of traditional Western and pelvic
theater and the way those conventions constitute power relationships. Both theaters are cultural constructions that are structured to help define proper performances and relationships. Although the pelvic theater that involves Gerry is
unique and while there is variation in each performance of a pelvic exam, understanding the conventions of traditional pelvic theater—the roles, set, props,
and so on that are ritually replayed with each exam—reveals the repetitive and
systematic components that codify pelvics.

Feminine Performativity and Pornography

Henslin and Biggs use a dramaturgical model to discount the uncooperative and
complaining patient as rare and disruptive to the optimal type of vaginal exam
performance. In other words, the authors purport that the pelvic exam performance structure as it exists is ideal, but the behavior of this particular patient,
Gerry, is the problem. Or rather, her performativity is the problem. Not only
does she reside in the troublesome position of a woman exposing her privates as
public spectacle, but she is making herself even more *spectacular* by "acting out."
    This staged quality of femininity which manifests itself in performative out-
bursts has been consistently pathologized within medicine. Gerry is great great
granddaughter to Charcot's nineteenth-century hysteric patients at Salpêtrière,
women whose treatment exemplifies the way the medical institution has associated femininity with pathology and performance. Hysteria, from the Latin *hysterus*, or uterus, was linked to females by way of their reproductive organs. Illness manifested itself in bodily performance, performance that even matched
acting styles of the period. The hysterics were presented in an amphitheater
where medical professionals (alongside actors and actresses) could observe
them.[8] As did the hysterics' outbursts for Charcot, Gerry's troublesome performativity provides observable and recordable research material for Henslin
and Biggs. However, while Charcot's hysterics were clothed, Gerry is not. Making public the pelvic patient's privates is always already in need of dramaturgical
regulation, according to Henslin and Biggs. But add to this display a spectacular
performativity, historically associated with pathological femininity, and the
outcome is especially volatile.
    Improper female performativity in the context of the vaginal exam could also

push the scene into the realm of the pornographic. By not properly playing the part of exam object, Gerry exercises a suggestive resistance and, in effect, heightens the situation's pornographic possibilities. This could be yet another reason why Henslin and Biggs place so much attention on proper female performance. The struggle between the apologetic mother, the resistant and sexually inexperienced daughter, the examining doctor, and the nurse-accomplice, who is referred to as both "pelvic preparer" and "chaperone," reads like a Sadeian narrative. Gerry has been surgically prepared for the impending loss of her virginity; the very nature of Gerry's pathology, her narrow opening demanding surgical widening in order to make way for a penis, is by itself highly overdetermined. The staging of the pelvic exam confirms her ability to perform the proper duties of a wife. The doctor checks out his handiwork—using the speculum as a diagnostic dildo—despite the cries and pain of the young girl. More perversely, he is supported by the encouraging mother and helpful nurse. In this narrative, not only is the pelvic exam preparation for the first sexual experience, it also reads like a first sexual experience in and of itself. The titillation of fear and pain, key ingredients of a Sadeian tale, establish an uncomfortable erotics.

The Seductive Patient

The flip side of a resistant woman patient like Gerry is the seductive patient; she is another favorite character who "acts out" in short porn narratives and medical anecdotes alike. The seductive patient is the woman who seeks out or eagerly welcomes examination in order to obtain pleasure. "The Seductive Patient" was the title of a 1982 article in *Medical Aspects of Human Sexuality*. A roundtable discussion among three male physicians warns other (male) physicians of the signs and threat of the woman patient who is a seductress. One physician advises: "I've observed some things that can serve as clues. For example, on repeated visits, the character of the patient's mode of dress may change, the clothes worn by the patient become more and more seductive and revealing—the low heels become high heels, more perfume is used, the makeup is put on differently—and become somewhat inappropriate for an appointment with a physician."[9] In this physician's schematic rendering of the seductive patient, the degree to which the patient *performs* femininity—how she costumes herself, how she applies makeup, the height of her heels—are the signs for which the physician must be on guard. An excessive display of femininity, deemed "inappropriate for an appointment with a physician," serves as the warning sign of a patient who is seductive. The physician's role as critic is expanded here: not only does he note biological pathologies, but also the possible pathological condition of "seductiveness." Implicitly, this roundtable discussion circulates around the male-physician/female-patient dyad that, along with its implicit focus on female sexuality, makes gynecology an obvious concern: "Gynecologists frequently encounter the overtly seductive patient and feel that this is peculiar to their specialty."[10] The article's frontispiece is a full-color print of a Mucha poster, picturing an archetypal "seductive woman" with low-neck gown, bare arms, long hair, half-closed eyes, and parted lips. The woman patient is cast as seductress, unable to contain herself at the prospect of bodily contact, threatening the properly "desexualized" medical exam.

Similarly, sociologist Joan Emerson in her article "Behavior in Private Places: Sustaining Definitions of Reality in Gynecological Examinations," locates the female patient as the troublemaker when it comes to challenging what she calls "reality in gynecological examinations." The appropriate "reality," according to Emerson, mirroring Henslin and Biggs, places the physician in the role of active examiner while the patient becomes the "technical object." According to Emerson, patients must be cooperative (allowing themselves to be technical object), but not overly cooperative (thus slipping into the category of seductive patient): "Some patients fail to know when to display their private parts unashamedly to others and when to conceal them like anyone else. A patient may make an 'inappropriate' show of modesty, thus not granting the staff the right to view what others do not. But if patients act as though they literally accept the medical definition this also constitutes a threat. If a patient insists on acting as if the exposure of her breasts, buttocks, and pelvic area are no different from exposure of her arm or leg, she is 'immodest.'"[11] An inappropriate public staging of the privates is the risk once again. And once again, it is the female patient's performance that is the focus of concern. Placed in the position of spectacle, the gynecological patient is always in something of a quandary. Since, by definition, the pelvic exam necessitates the highly overdetermined and anxiety-producing acts of female genital exposure and manipulation, a great deal of attention has been displaced onto how the patient "acts," onto *her* performance.

Theatrical language was employed by these sociologists in order to define what constituted proper performance for female patients. Rather than question attitudes about female genital display and manipulation, the authors made the female patient scapegoat for cultural anxieties surrounding gynecology, female bodies, sexuality, and genitals. Is it simply a coincidence that these articles appeared contemporaneously with the rise of feminism and the women's health movement? As more and more women were asserting the importance of being active performers in the management of their bodies and health, particularly with regard to their reproductive organs, these researchers were defining the proper boundaries of pelvic theater, stressing the importance of disciplined role play that positioned women patients as passive and compliant. Theatrical terms were not used in order to *critique* power or gender relationships within the pelvic exam scenario, but rather to *enforce, naturalize,* and *essentialize* the performance of those prescribed roles.

The Sacred Vagina

In concluding this analysis, we shall briefly indicate that conceptualizing the vagina as a sacred object yields a perspective that appears to be of value in analyzing the vaginal examination. —Henslin and Biggs, "Dramaturgical Desexualization"

At the close of their essay, Henslin and Biggs propose that the "vagina as a sacred object" has certain rules governing who may approach it (husband and physician) and under what circumstances. In a footnote they declare, "It is perhaps for this reason that prostitutes ordinarily lack respect: they have profaned the sacred."[12] The vagina is constructed as somehow separate from the woman herself. Her vagina is inherently sacred; the woman is not. Rather it is her duty to present her vagina in the correct fashion and to the right public. The authors offer this reasoning as a justification for their attention to proper female performance. The medical institution is constructed as champion of this sacred vagina, simultaneously protecting it from the profanity of disease while performatively protecting it from the profanity of improper interactions: "the ritual of the vaginal examination allows the doctor to approach the sacred without profaning it or violating taboos by dramaturgically defining the vagina as just another organ of the body, disassociating the vagina from the person, while desexualizing the person into a cooperative object."[13] According to Henslin and Biggs, the vagina is sacred, revered by the medical establishment, whereas the woman herself is made into little more than a "cooperative object," thus privileging the drama that occurs between the woman's legs and its accompanying roles over the drama that occurs backstage.

But this insistence that the vagina is essentially "sacred" is suspicious given the many ways in which the vagina is otherwise culturally rendered "profane" (menstruation taboos, vaginal "odor," vagina dentata, etc.). The vagina's marginality, the fact that it links the outside and the inside of the body, and the ways that it incorporates qualities from both spheres help give the vagina its reputation as a charged zone: the vagina sports moist, textured tissues like bodily insides while it is accessible from the outside without an incision. In the terms of anthropologist Mary Douglas, the vagina is not inherently "pure" or sacred, but is potentially dangerous and in danger of entering the "profane" by virtue of its very marginality.[14] In her analysis of the female nude in visual art, Lynda Nead notes, "The forms, conventions and poses of art have worked metaphorically to shore up the female body—to seal orifices and to prevent marginal matter from transgressing the boundary dividing the inside of the body and the outside, the self from the space of the other."[15] In the classic female nude, the vagina is sealed and the vulva is rendered as smooth surface, containing female excess and sexuality. The pelvic exam implicitly contradicts this contained and containing representation. Through the pelvic exam, the clinician encounters openings, secretions, and ridged surfaces (known as vaginal rugae). In pelvic examinations, specifically the introduction of the speculum or clinician fingers into the vagina, boundaries are transgressed. The space between the self and the other to which Nead refers is momentarily collapsed. Thus, although it resides in continual negotiation with the classical body, the female pelvic patient's body more aptly fits the definition of the grotesque body[16]—a body with excessive orifices and fluids.

Henslin and Biggs's almost casual assumption that the vagina is culturally defined as "sacred" as explanation for dramaturgical desexualization is reductive and naive. This assumption, in keeping with their desire to essentialize and naturalize female behavior and bodies, legitimates a theatricalized objectification (literally, making object) of the woman patient within the pelvic exam on the basis of the importance of *maintaining* the sacredness of the vagina during the pelvic exam performance. Rather, in representation and practice the vulva and vagina are continually being negotiated, oscillating between the poles (limiting as binaries are) of sacred-profane, classical-grotesque, pure-dangerous. While the transformation of the woman patient into a cooperative object within the pelvic exam is explained as a move to protect the vagina as sacred object, it is instead an attempt to contain those threatening qualities that constitute the female body as profane, grotesque, and dangerous.

The Drape-Sheet Screen

According to Henslin and Biggs, Gerry resisted the role of uncomplaining object. With her discomfort, anxiety, and other more vocal performative outbursts, she was fairly successful in stealing center stage from her "sacred" vagina. However, the structures of the pelvic exam continued to position Gerry, as they do many other women, as passive object of examination while treating her vagina as though it were disembodied. Consider the use of posters or images plastered on gynecological exam room ceilings that are meant to occupy or entertain women as they receive exams. Consider the way that some practitioners attempt to distract patients with talk about anything nongynecological and how others will not speak at all. In interviews I conducted, numerous women recalled feeling absent during their exams: "leaving my body on the table," "retreating into my head," and "being made to feel invisible." Even though their very visible, living bodies were on the exam table, these women expressed a feeling of absence or invisibility. These sentiments suggest that relationships between players in the pelvic exam production are more complicated than conventional understandings of theater may permit. For instance, theorist Christian Metz used the very terms "presence" and "absence" when discussing differences between spectatorship in the theater and the cinema: "In the theater, actors and spectators are present at the same time and in the same location, hence present one to another, as the two protagonists of an authentic perverse couple. But in the cinema, the actor was present when the spectator was not (=shooting), and the spectator is present when the actor is no longer (=projection): a failure to meet of the voyeur and the exhibitionist whose approaches no longer coincide (they have 'missed' one another)."[17] If we consider the gynecological practitioner to be spectator and woman patient to be actress, the description of cinematic spectatorship is a more fitting model for considering those women who are rendered absent during an exam. It is as though the drape sheet is the screen, dividing the woman's pelvic region from the rest of her body; anything behind the screen can then be treated as nonexistent.

In her book *The Woman in the Body*, Emily Martin cites an interview with a woman she calls Eileen Miller who shares similar feelings about her birthing experience: "Oftentimes when you're having a baby the doctors act like they're watching TV. Your legs are up and you're draped and all of them are going like this [gestures in the air with a poking motion]. You wonder what they have down there, a portable TV, or are they really working on me?"[18] Miller's description of her birthing experience could certainly be referring to the increasing technologization of birth (e.g., use of fetal monitors) and the use of anesthetics that numb from the waist down (e.g., epidurals). But the idea of a TV between her legs represents the ways in which medical—specifically gynecologic and obstetric—technologies and structures can leave the (absent) female patient behind the screen, placing the clinician in the position of distanced spectator. When patients like Gerry attempt to dismantle the screen by asserting their own positions as spectators, they are offered as examples of uncompliant, inappropriate, and troublesome patients.

Such institutionalized absence as that located within the pelvic exam and birthing scenarios complicates Christian Metz's straightforward notion of experiential presence and representational absence in theater and film spectatorship.

While, in Metz's terms, both clinician and patient are *present* during the performance of the exam, the woman patient can be made *absent*. Metz's *presence* and *absence* elide the fact that theater and performance, like film and television, are also mediated forms. Likewise, medicine is a blending of the filmic and theatric economies. The medical apparatus, with its attendant technologies and modes of vision, addresses live bodies, but the effects of this apparatus upon the patient-subject, particularly the pelvic subject, may in effect render her *absent*. Theater and performance theorists such as Jill Dolan have invested a great deal in maintaining the *presence* of the female performer.[19] However, this is not always possible within the performance of the traditional pelvic exam because the female patient-performer's *presence* is often carefully mediated. Absence in gynecology is not simply a physical absolute, but is created by a system that frequently dissociates women from their bodies, making them into "pelvis[es]-that-incidentally-belong-to-[people]." Even though Gerry insisted on asserting her presence throughout her exam, we will consider what the results of her rebellion really were and whether such performative *presence* actually paid off given the structures that were in place.

Gendered Spectatorship

Riddle: A boy and his father were in a car accident. The father was killed. The boy
is brought into the operating room and the surgeon proclaims "This is my son!"
How can this be?

In Gerry's pelvic performance, it is expected that the physician is in complete control and that the young woman patient remain passive and accepting. The fact that Gerry is young and female and the physician examining her is male is left undiscussed by Henslin and Biggs: the underlying assumption, and the statistical probability at the time Henslin and Biggs wrote their article, was that the physician would be male. But this gendering of the two players no doubt inflects the performance in specific ways. Imagine if Gerry were a young man receiving a male genital exam and the physician a woman. The race of the two players is also left unspecified. Imagine if Gerry were a young African American female and the physician white or, if Gerry were white and her physician African American. How then would the performance have been framed? But because race is not mentioned, whiteness is assumed and, for Henslin and Biggs, the gender of the participating practitioner is unremarkable as well.

The riddle that opens this section plays on the gendered assumptions regarding physicians, particularly surgeons. How can the boy be the surgeon's son if the father was killed? Answer: The surgeon is the boy's mother. Assumptions regarding the gender of the physician are historically grounded. Only recently have women played a statistically significant role in modern medicine. Whereas the physician-spectator who maintains the scientific and medical gaze is traditionally gendered male, the object of that gaze is gendered female. In her book *Sexual Visions*, Ludmilla Jordanova traces this gendered spectator-spectacle relationship to eighteenth-century images in science and medicine. In such images, the scientific and medical gaze was male and the female body symbolized nature. Thus the imaging of the female body, its continual unveiling and dissection in practice and representation, signified *man's* scientific search for the essence of nature.[20] Giuliana Bruno makes a similar claim for cinema: "Just as the anatomical gaze, the cinematic gaze 'dissects' by moving across and in depth, plunging into space and traversing it."[21] Bruno connects the history of the cinema with an anatomical curiosity and, like Jordanova, locates the object of the gaze as women's anatomy. Thus "cinema's analytic genealogically descends, in a way, from a distinct anatomic fascination for the woman's body."[22] This fascination stems from a preoccupation with otherness in relation to the male body, established as norm; it is coupled with a pathologization of female bodily difference. Laura Mulvey is attributed with first suggesting the way in which cinema, particularly classical Hollywood narrative cinema, produces a viewing subject that is active and gendered male, while the object of the gaze, "the bearer of the look," is passive, pathologized, and gendered female.[23] Henslin and Biggs assigned these very same roles to model players in the pelvic theater. It is as though they were not only attempting to locate the ideal pelvic exam, but also the ideal Hollywood screenplay. But whereas their descriptions of the ideal pelvic exam were a move toward the *desexualization* of the female gynecological spectacle, their description when applied to cinematic spectatorship is the same formula applied to the *sexualization* of the female cinematic spectacle.

Historically, this gendered spectator-spectacle relationship mirrors the gendered gynecological exam in which traditionally there is an active male physician-spectator and a passive female patient-spectacle. And, parallel to Mulvey's analysis of the male spectator, the male physician, in accordance with popular gynecological discourse, has been attributed a certain degree of unconscious scopophilic, voyeuristic (even sadistic) pleasure. For this reason, John M. Smith, M.D., a practicing gynecologist for more than fifteen years, states in his popular book *Women and Doctors*, "After years of closely observing the personalities and behavior of [male] gynecologists, I have to conclude that for many the subconscious motivation may involve the need to be in a powerful and controlling relationship with women."[24] His main suggestion for change is to increase the number of female gynecologists,[25] the assumption being that the introduction of an active *female* spectator within the gynecology apparatus would thereby change the relationship between spectator and spectacle.[26]

But does simply plugging more women into gynecology in its traditional form necessarily make change? Would Gerry's script or Henslin and Biggs's conclusions have been decidedly different if the physician had been female? Mulvey's analysis is helpful here. In her important essay "Visual Pleasure and Narrative Cinema," the possibility of a "woman in the audience" is almost completely disavowed. In her formulation the cinematic apparatus, like the gynecological apparatus in Henslin and Biggs's formulation, simply structures and positions all spectators as male.[27] However, in a subsequent essay, "Afterthoughts on 'Visual Pleasure and Narrative Cinema' inspired by King Vidor's *Duel in the Sun* (1946)," Mulvey rethinks the possibility of a female spectator. The female spectator, according to Mulvey, is refigured as still having a "masculine point of view," but one to which she has an uneasy relationship. The female spectator is left "shifting between the metaphoric opposition 'active' and 'passive.' "[28] This position of the female spectator in cinema is helpful in considering the position of the female gynecologist who must similarly oscillate between identifying with the passive female patient on the table (with whom she shares anatomy and the experience of playing pelvic patient) and with the position of the active male physician (with whom she shares certain privileges with regard to the medical gaze and power). But her split between these two positions may be weighted more in one direction than the other. There may seem to be more advantages to identifying with the position of active male physician in terms of status, money, and so on than with the female patient. Likewise, institutional factors such as a female physician's training and role models may further influence her close identification with the former position.

Mary Ann Doane's discussion of women's films of the 1940s that include doctor-patient scenarios is useful in considering the subject position of the female gynecologist. Doane notes that "the films of the medical discourse encourage the female spectator to repudiate the feminine pole and to ally herself with the one who diagnoses, with a medical gaze."[29] When the medical and cinematic spheres are collapsed in the body of the medical discourse film, Doane finds that the female spectator is encouraged to identify with the active male medical gaze over the passive pathological female patient. In medical practice, there is an expectation that a woman physician would readily identify with her female patient. In interviews, many women have expressed astonishment over a negative experience with a female clinician. How could a woman treat them poorly or roughly? Given the implicit hierarchies of the clinic, medical pedagogy, and medical and broader cultural attitudes toward women and women's bodies, the gynecological apparatus helps construct gynecologists', even female gynecologists', attitudes toward female bodies.

There are limitations to Mulvey's analysis for cinema and therefore its application to gynecology. Psychoanalysis dictates the cinematic experience (e.g., the types of identification) available for the gendered spectator. To the extent that they have control over their own subjectivity and agency, spectators may offer resistant readings, identifying in ways not predicted by gaze theory. Just as there are female and male spectators who have resisted their implied subject positions within the cinematic apparatus, there are compassionate female and male gynecologists who have differently negotiated the traditional gynecological apparatus. But all too often both unconsciously and consciously the subject position proposed by the apparatus is accepted; many male gynecologists, as well as female gynecologists, have readily adopted the ideology of the apparatus, partaking of misogynist modes of practice that situate women patients as passive objects of the gaze and female sexuality as pathological.

I do not mean that gynecology, or any other medicalized form of women or men looking at women's genitals, is inherently flawed. I recognize, as Laura Kipnis points out, that the term "the male gaze" has become an overused monolith among critics that carries with it the possible assumption that men looking is bad and that whatever men look at is "objectified."[30] As Kipnis argues, this certainly does not take into account the differing power that men (and women) have, nor does it account for race and ethnicity, which play an important structural function within a cinematic (and gynecological) apparatus. Undoubtedly, the race of the clinician also influences his or her relationship to the gynecological apparatus, just as the *perceived* race of the patient frames the physician's analysis. The race or ethnicity of the patient has historically coded her body, guiding how it is viewed and, therefore, how it is diagnosed. For example, there have traditionally been "white women's" pelvic diseases (e.g., endometriosis) and "black women's" diseases (e.g., pelvic inflammatory disease). These are not empirically based distinctions, rather they are dependent on cultural stereotypes regarding race and pathology.

Gynecology has traditionally been heterosexist as well, denying the possibility of participants who are not heterosexual. Mulvey's initial theory is predominantly heteronormative and does not account for gay, lesbian, or bisexual identities. Within Mulvey's scenario, the proposed spectator is heterosexual and male; the proposed "bearer of the look" is heterosexual and female. How is a gay male clinician incorporated into (or excluded from) the gynecological apparatus? a lesbian practitioner? a lesbian patient? More and more critical work in both film and theater addresses gay and lesbian subjectivity in relation to performance and cinematic texts.[31] The heteronormativity of traditional gynecology, a practice that, for instance, almost always assumes all its patients are heterosexually active, continually needs to be challenged as well.[32] Queer theorists' contributions to considerations of cinema and theater and performance spectatorship can help call into question the heteronormativity of medical, specifically gynecological, practice and representation.

Looking Back

With regard to spectatorship, most of the attention in film theory has been focused on the position of the audience-spectator. However, the gynecological gaze can be theorized in both directions. Not only does the clinician look at the patient, but the patient can also look back at the clinician. In Gerry's case, not only was she the center of attention, but she too was experiencing her own examination, observing the physician, her mother, and the nurse. How can the patient-spectacle look back within the pelvic exam and how can we consider this look? This "looking back" has been particularly significant within the theorization of theater and performance. Peggy Phelan's notion of the "potential reciprocal gaze" elegantly locates this possibility within performance and theater as well as within other representational media: photographs, paintings, films, and political protests.[33] Engaging Bertolt Brecht as foundational to Mulvey's analysis of cinema as well as to new formulations regarding the female performer and the female spectator of theater and performance, Elin Diamond asserts that the actor-subject is "theoretically free to look back."[34] Diamond draws on Brecht in order to theorize "a female body in representation that resists fetishization and a viable position for the female spectator," recognizing that it is "Brechtian intervention that signals a way of dismantling the gaze."[35] Through distanciation, the actor-subject distances herself from the character she portrays so that she does not "impersonate" the character but rather "demonstrates" or "quotes" her behavior.

Is such distanciation viable for the pelvic patient-subject? May she distance herself from her role as pelvic patient in order to comment on the ideology of the gynecological exam? In Gerry's case, the very "looking back" and "acting out" that constituted her resistance to the proper role of pelvic patient could be viewed as a Brechtian performance. She demonstrated improper behavior rather than impersonating the proper pelvic object. However, given the encompassing gynecological apparatus, this distanciation only served to further pathologize Gerry. Thus Gerry's performativity, the very behavior that Diamond might regard as resisting fetishization of the female body, resulted in a more furtive fetishization and pathologization. Thus it must be highlighted that the stakes are different for Gerry than for a Brechtian stage performer. Her actions may be better understood as a reaction to her immediate situation than as premeditated political performance. For Gerry, distanciation is not necessarily a chosen mode of performance, but one in which she partakes because of limited options.

Due to the larger cultural and medical apparatus, Gerry is damned if she does and damned if she doesn't. If she *does* behave properly, collapsing actor-subject and character, she will be accepting her place within an apparatus in which she is a priori defined as pathological due to her gender and anatomy. If she *does not* behave properly, engaging in a Brechtian resistance that points to the separation between actor-subject and character, her performative resistance will still result in her pathologization. Her behavior is deemed problematic by her physician, who must now have a long talk with her, and by Henslin and Biggs, who locate her performance as inappropriate. Thus Diamond's model might be a bit too optimistic in considering possibilities for an actor-subject like Gerry.

However, Diamond's attempt to locate a viable position for the female spectator through a consideration of Brechtian interventions may be more applicable here with regard to the critic-spectator. According to Diamond's model, the spectator may distinguish between the actor-subject and the character. With regard to the pelvic exam, the critic may distinguish between the female patient and the role she is positioned to play. This does not locate the spectator-critic as either outside of representation or privileged due to her particular identity. Nor are all critic-spectators able to distinguish between the actor-subject and character. For instance, Biggs, the coauthor of "Dramaturgical Desexualization," served as a critic-spectator, using her experience as a gynecological nurse as fodder for her academic writings oriented at keeping women performing in passive and compliant ways. However, in recognizing this distance between actor-subject and character, Diamond's critic-spectator may ideally be able to reformulate scripts, stagings, and characters. In order to reformulate them, it is first important to understand the stagings, roles, and scripts that constitute the gynecological apparatus, to consider the play between these structures and the agencies of the subjects performing. Such reformulations are made possible through critical analyses of the ways the pelvic exam is performed and the structures that underlie it.

Apparatus and Performance

The term "apparatus," as I have used it above, is important to this consideration of the pelvic exam as performance. In his essay "Ideological Effects of the Basic

Cinematographic Apparatus," Jean-Louis Baudry employs psychoanalysis to propose that the instruments or "technical base" (camera, screen, etc.) of the cinema are simultaneously overdetermined by and productive of dominant ideology.[36] The term "apparatus" allows for a much broader consideration of cinema in relation to culture than its mechanics. As Philip Rosen notes: "Thus, as often as not, when the apparatus is theorized, the writer will have in mind not simply 'the cinema machine' in a literal sense (e.g. the basic camera-projector mechanism), but this literal machine in the context of a larger social and/or cultural and/or institutional 'machine,' for which the former is only a point of convergence of several lines of force of the latter."[37] In discussing the apparatus of the pelvic exam, many cultural and technological aspects may be considered: the literal "machine" of the exam (e.g., speculum, drape sheet, exam table, clinician, patient, space of the exam room, positionality of clinician and patient, etc.), the many ways in which gynecology and pelvic exams enter into a broader social and/or cultural machine (e.g., popular film and performance art), and how the institutional medicine machine (e.g., medical pedagogy, medical history, medical textbooks) comes into play.[38] My uneasiness with psychoanalysis as an explanatory narrative for the apparatus leads me from Baudry to Foucault, whose notion of the apparatus is in many ways analogous, but avoids the pitfalls of Freud and Lacan. On the term "apparatus," Foucault notes: "What I'm trying to pick out with this term is, firstly, a thoroughly heterogenous ensemble consisting of discourses, institutions, architectural forms, regulatory decisions, laws, administrative measures, scientific statements, philosophical, moral and philanthropic propositions—in short the said as much as the unsaid. Such are the elements of the apparatus. The apparatus itself is the system of relations that can be established between these elements . . . The apparatus is thus always inscribed in a play of power, but it is also always linked to certain coordinates of knowledge which issue from it but, to an equal degree, condition it."[39]

The notion of an apparatus allows for a consideration of everyday life practices, the play between overdetermined structures within representations and practices and what Michel deCerteau calls "the ways in which users operate," the tactics employed by everyday life consumers-producers-performers.[40] Everyday life performers simultaneously negotiate and are negotiated by the "heterogenous ensemble" that constitutes an apparatus. This calls into question the manner in which some theorists have singled out performance as a particularly privileged theoretical principle or modality for critical analysis. For example, in *Unmarked*, Phelan maintains that performance is "representation without reproduction."[41] Part of the difficulty here is that Phelan slips in and out of talking about performance generally, as in everyday life, and staged performance, specifically performance art and theater. While there are instances for which this distinction is unclear (e.g., the "life performance" work of Linda Montano)[42] and while there are sometimes good political reasons for preventing any clear distinction, Phelan's theorizations consistently conflate the two. By not making this distinction, one runs the risk of attaching complete volition and therefore agency to an individual's performance in everyday life, regardless of socioeconomic, cultural, and institutional factors.

Phelan argues that, "Without a copy, live performance plunges into visibility—in a maniacally charged present—and disappears into memory, into the realm of invisibility and the unconscious where it eludes regulation and control."[43] She states that, with performance "there are no left-overs," rather it is "completely consumed." This affords performance, in her terms, a unique power: "Performance's independence from mass reproduction, technologically, economically, and linguistically, is its greatest strength."[44] What modality or medium *is* simultaneously representation and reproduction? A consideration of representations and practices fitting into a larger apparatus challenges Phelan's claim. For example, while there may be two material copies of the same film, the situation in which the film is shown, the audience, the manner in which it is viewed, and so on continually shift. No representation is thoroughly reproducible in this sense; each enters into a new set of relations with its encompassing apparatus of reception and interpretation.

Likewise, performance does not operate within a completely contained and consumable economy. As is evident in the many performances of gynecology examined throughout this book, there are indeed "left-overs," performance traces that influence and in turn are influenced by numerous other representations and practices. In this sense, performance is no more pure or unmediated than any other representational practice. Performance is inherently neither more natural nor less technological than other media. Moreover, both staged and everyday life performance are in continual negotiation with other technologies and media. Contrary to Phelan's claims, mass reproduction is saturated by performance (consider the performativity of the assembly line) and performance by mass reproduction.[45] Phelan is interested in "the politics of performance," but her theoretical model risks *depoliticizing* performance by extricating ideology and power from it in order to make the idea and medium of performance more "purely" powerful.

By invoking the term "performance," I do not assert the superiority or primacy of performance as a theoretical model. Rather, I turn to performance in order to bridge two normally segregated areas: practice and representation. This segregation is particularly evident with regard to medicine: the contemporary *practice* of examination is scrutinized by social scientists and medical professionals, while medical *representation* (historical, visual, literary, etc.) is analyzed primarily by theorists in the humanities. In highlighting the staged quality of practice, it becomes clear that pelvic exam practice is itself representational, reflecting underlying ideas about female bodies, pathology, sexuality, sex, and gender, as in the case of Gerry. Likewise, investigations of representations such as sociological cases, medical textbook images, performance art, and historical texts as performative practices reveal that representations impact and reflect everyday life practices. Thus, employing the term "performance," which simultaneously refers to a *practiced act* and a *constructed representation*, is an attempt to critique the representation-practice divide and the limits it has placed on critics.

In Gerry's case, a consideration of the performance apparatus allows for a consideration of the many ways in which ideology, power, spectatorship, pathology, gender, and sex come into play within the framework of the pelvic exam. Her story reveals that the pelvic exam is a constitutive performance that is highly productive with regard to gender and the materiality of sex. Unlike Emerson and Henslin and Biggs, I do not use performance terms in order to reiterate the "proper" behavior for the female spectacle. Rather, beginning with the case of Gerry and following with a variety of historical and contemporary practices and representations, I attempt to locate as well as critique one of many "heterogenous ensembles" that constitutes the performance apparatus of the pelvic exam, to show the interrelation between this heterogenous ensemble and other cultural structures, and to suggest possible alternative structures and ways of changing the apparatus. The focus must shift from Gerry's performance and from what constitutes a proper performance for the female patient. The apparatus must accommodate more than two options for the female patient—that she exhibits either proper passive behavior or misbehavior in the form of acting out. There needs to be a consideration of what it means to be patient, spectacle, spectator, director, and performer in the pelvic theater.

2 Mastering the Female Pelvis:
Race and the Tools of Reproduction

And if in these days a moment can be spared for sentimental reverie, look again,
I beg, at the curious speculum, and gazing through the confused reflections from
its bright curves, catch a fleeting glimpse of an old hut in Alabama and seven negro
women who suffered, and endured, and had rich reward. —J. Chassar Moir, M.D.,
The Vesico-Vaginal Fistula[1]

During the four years between 1845 and 1849, J. Marion Sims, M.D., conducted
surgical experiments on slave women in his backyard hospital in Montgomery,
Alabama. These women all had vesico-vaginal fistulas, small tears that form
between the vagina and urinary tract or bladder which cause urine to leak un-
controllably. Through repeated surgeries, Sims attempted to repair the fistulas.
He is now remembered as the Father of American Gynecology, Father of Modern Gynecology, and Architect of the Vagina. Following the eventual success of
the surgical reparation, Sims won illustrious titles, awards, and fame worldwide and praising words in most contemporary gynecology and medical history texts.[2] By his own estimation he became "the second wealthiest of all
American physicians."[3] As we shall see, Sims's fame and wealth are as indebted
to slavery and racism as they are to innovation, insight, and persistence, and he
has left behind a frightening legacy of medical attitudes toward and treatments

of women, particularly women of color. These four years of surgical experimentation on slave women represent the foundation of gynecology as a distinct specialty.

Through an investigation of Sims's practices, a number of important distinctions regarding the foundation of gynecology will become clear. First, the institution of slavery served medicine in providing subjects for experimentation. The gynecological patients' position as slaves defined their status as medical subjects, situating them as institutionally powerless and therefore as fitting props for the experimenting white physician-turned-master-showman, who revealed, probed, and operated on their vaginas. Slavery enabled the foundation of gynecology and in the process helped define the proper object of medical experimentation.

Second, the use of the speculum in North America was founded on slave women's bodies. This medical precedent prompts questions that will be asked throughout this book: What kind of woman is considered to be most appropriate for speculum examination? How does gynecological display structure physician-patient power differentials? The position of Sims's patients as slaves made them more fitting objects for speculum penetration and the physician's gaze while, at the same time, their status as slaves was reiterated by the physician's probing gaze and penetrating speculum as tools of medical discipline. An investigation of this historic medical innovation provides insight into the way gynecology continues to situate patients.

Third, Sims's surgical experimentation set a precedent for the medical institution's involvement in racist, eugenicist practices concerned with the reproductive capacities of poor women of color. His surgical reparation can be viewed as an early reproductive technology aimed at helping to optimize the reproductive capacity of slave capital. In a welfare state economy, reproductive technologies to foster pregnancy are often marketed at wealthy, predominantly white women, whereas new technologies aimed at limiting reproduction are most often used experimentally on poor women of color and subsequently aimed at them through accessibility and legislated incentives. Norplant, a surgically implanted contraceptive, will be investigated as technological offspring to Sims's surgical reparation of vesico-vaginal fistulas. This association does not assume or assert that either technology is inherently "bad," but rather points to the ways in which technological innovation and use are generated by and help reinforce ideological structures, including institutionalized racism. Thus an investigation of Sims's practices provides a look at foundational moments in gynecology. Racism, slavery, and the thrill of medical innovation were all joined in the early days of the discipline. Their reverberations are still felt today.

Master Showman

As a historical player, Sims is key to a consideration of the relationship between performance and gynecology. In fact, performance is often enlisted as an explanatory model for Sims's behavior. In his autobiography, eulogies following his death, and a biography published in 1950, Sims is rhetorically positioned as a sensational surgical performer. His patients, however, are situated as passive, proplike objects rather than co-performers. By simply orchestrating the unveiling of the previously mysterious internal landscape of the live female pelvis, Sims gained vast fame and devoted followers, and his dramatic surgeries cemented his reputation as a master showman. Early in his career, he performed to a small audience of eager physicians in his makeshift backyard hospital, but later he played to larger and larger crowds at the Woman's Hospital in New York as well as in famous operating theaters abroad.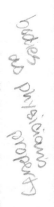

Seale Harris, M.D., Sims's biographer and the son of one of his disciples, notes, "Sims had a great love for the theater and everything dramatic, and he was fascinated by P. T. Barnum's combination of master showmanship (for which he himself had a not inconsiderable gift)." In his autobiography, Sims mentions "spending time with my good friend Mr. P. T. Barnum" in the summer of 1849 in New Orleans.[4] What might link a surgeon-slave-master to a showman-ringmaster? Both exercise mastery over bodies, particularly grotesque bodies (in the sense of either open, oozing bodies or freaks). The high drama of surgery, like the daring circus feat, demands courage in order to perform that which seems impossible. And both the ringmaster and the surgeon-slave-master perform to large audiences, commanding center stage.[5]

Barnum's shows and exhibits were simultaneously science, art, education, and entertainment. Oftentimes, ambiguities in race and even species served as the titillating freakishness for his exhibits. For instance, the Leopard Child, a young boy with vitiligo, a condition that causes abnormal pigmentation, was a "favorite with spectators at the American Museum."[6] William Henry Johnson, an African American known as "Zip," was exhibited in Barnum's Gallery of Wonders as a missing link, that could be a "lower order of man" or a "higher order of monkey."[7]

Of special interest is Joice Heth, "a blind, decrepit, hymn-singing" slave woman for whom Barnum purchased "the right to exhibit." He claimed Heth was 161 years old and had been nurse to George Washington.[8] Before her death, Barnum promised Dr. David L. Rogers, "an eminent New York surgeon who had examined Joice upon her first arrival in the metropolis, that he would have the opportunity to dissect her should she die while under Barnum's management."[9]

When the time came, there gathered "a large crowd of physicians, medical students, clergymen, and (naturally) editors, each of whom was assessed fifty cents for this extraordinary privilege." In the end, the surgeon found that Heth was not even eighty.

What is freakish is not the boy with vitiligo or the slave women with vesico-vaginal fistulas. Rather, the true atrocities are the methods enlisted to display the "freaks" and the atrocious types of intervention used. Both Sims's and Barnum's spectacles were consistently fashioned as simultaneously passive, proplike freaks and uncontrolled bodies in need of taming. Though one commanded center stage in a hospital and the other in a circus, what links Sims and Barnum is a fascination with difference, ambiguity, and pathology, a fascination that is premised on race, power, and exhibition. And visibility.

The Fistula

Sims did not plan to found his career on "disorders peculiar to women." In his autobiography, *The Story of My Life*, he admits, "If there was anything I hated, it was investigating the organs of the female pelvis."[10] Yet "women's problems" seemed to court him in his small general practice. He was repeatedly confronted with one particular condition: the vesico-vaginal fistula. Often a result of hard and extended childbirth, fistulas are what Sims referred to as "the sloughing of the soft parts."

Although white women also developed fistulas, when slaves developed them they were often blamed for not having called on white male physicians during difficult labor: "the [slave] women preferred to suffer in seclusion than to call for help at such time."[11] As Elizabeth Fox-Genovese notes in *Within the Plantation Household*, slaves largely distrusted white doctors, preferring black "root doctors" and herbal remedies, reflecting "African as well as local folk beliefs."[12] Elaborate systems of care were in place in many slave communities, providing slaves with treatments preferable to what they must have viewed as the dangerous practices upheld by the growing white male medical establishment at that time. But lay practitioners, particularly black ones, were systematically denounced by physicians who relegated them to the realm of malpractice. In a eulogy for Sims, one physician recounted, Sims "was not slow in finding cases of this disgusting disease, particularly among the slave population, whose management in accouchement was generally confined to the ignorant midwives of their own colour."[13] A favorite target of white male physicians, black midwives were held responsible for the slaves' vesico-vaginal fistulas.

Almost two-thirds of Montgomery's population at that time was slaves.

Sims's participation in the institution of slavery is explained in his biography: "The Simses themselves owned a number of Negroes. . . . It was the only way that they knew, and to them it seemed a good one."[14] Sims even purchased a slave expressly for the purpose of experimentation when her master resisted Sims's solicitations. Certainly the prevailing institution of slavery afforded Sims an opportune scenario in which to operate. Sims was then construed as their savior, an "evangelist of healing to women," who could no longer turn his back on these helpless sufferers.[15] Part of this messianic role included rescuing them from the "mis-management" of their own midwives.

Sims did not initially accept the challenge of the fistula. A slave master contacted him to check on a slave named Anarcha who had been in labor for three days. Sims proceeded to remove the baby with a forceps. All seemed to be fine with the woman, but five days later Sims found an extensive fistula that caused her to leak both urine and bowel. He had never before seen this condition and initially considered it a "surgical curiosity." Later, after reexamining the literature and finding that the condition had been noted but no physician had ever successfully repaired it, he explained to the woman's master that there was no hope of mending the fistula. In his autobiography, Sims recreates his words to the master: "Anarcha has an affliction that unfits her for the duties required of a servant. She will not die, but she will never get well, and all you have to do is to take good care of her so long as she lives."[16]

Here, Sims's first concern is Anarcha's ability to work. How would the fistula have made the slave unfit for her duties? While the fistula made this woman smell of bowel and urine, it would not have diminished her strength or ability to work. Sims's comment could be a reference to the fact that slave women were viewed as the "breeding" property of their masters. The slave's "duties" may refer not only to her labor as a slave in terms of work in the fields or house, but also to her sexual and reproductive duties: "Owners had a financial interest in slaves producing children and openly encouraged 'breeding.' Women known as breeders brought higher prices on the slave market and might enjoy special privileges, such as a job in the master's house rather than in the fields."[17] With this "disgusting disease" the slave would no longer be attractive or fit, thereby affecting her reproductive labor as a woman who would bear future slave labor. As Deborah Gray White asserts, "The perpetuation of the institution of slavery, as nineteenth century Southerners knew it, rested on the slave woman's reproductive capacity."[18] Viewing black female bodies as capital, slave owners found this bothersome condition troubling indeed. In addition, slave women were frequently approached as receptacles of white male sexual power: white men "expected to exercise sexual freedom with women slaves. Especially within the planter class, relations with black women provided white men with both a sexual outlet and a means of maintaining racial dominance."[19] The smell of urine and bowel would undoubtedly undermine this particular means of maintaining power over slave women.[20]

Masters were not unfamiliar with slave women being unfit for their duties because of their reproductive organs. And slave women sometimes used the knowledge that masters were particularly invested in their reproductive abilities to their advantage. A number of historians of slavery have noted evidence that some slave women feigned illness related to their reproductive organs, "playing the lady," as it was called, in order to temporarily diminish or eliminate their workload.[21] By "playing the lady," slave women were performing white womanhood, enlisting illness as a mode of resistance in order to manipulate their white masters' historically situated fears regarding the delicate and unpredictable female reproductive organs so vital to the masters' profits. In the case of "playing the lady," we find, as we did in the previous chapter in relation to Charcot's hysterics and the sociologists' hymenotomy patient, that femininity, performativity, pathology, and the reproductive organs are frequently thought to be interdependent.

Some masters were unsympathetic to slave women's illnesses, feigned or otherwise, and created various performances of their own that discouraged such resistance. As White notes, "Some masters insisted on giving the 'patient' a thorough examination before excusing her from work."[22] A slave who was "playing the lady" could potentially be faced with a master "playing doctor," a power-laden sexual and fact-finding threat. However, illness affecting slave women's reproductive labor was not taken lightly because it seriously threatened a master's earnings. Physicians such as Sims were called on to help when it was found that indeed the slave woman was not simply "playing."

About a month after Anarcha's examination, another slave woman, Betsey, was sent to Sims for inspection because she could not hold urine. She too had a fistula, and Sims sent her back to her master, explaining that he could do nothing. One month following Betsey's visit, Sims was contacted by a master whose slave, Lucy, had the same symptoms as Betsey. Despite Sims's protest that the master need not bother sending the woman, Lucy was sent and indeed, upon examination, was found to have a fistula. Sims gave her a bed in his homemade backyard hospital for "Negroes," but he informed her she had to leave the following afternoon. In his autobiography he wrote: "She was very much disappointed, for her condition was loathsome, and she was in hope that she could be cured."[23] Thus, in the autobiography, the stage is rhetorically set for the entrance of willing experimentees.

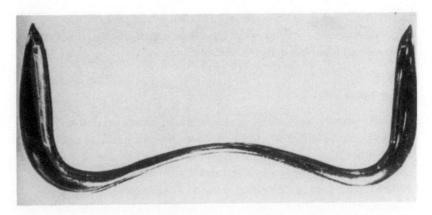

Figure 1. Sims's Speculum. In Emil Novak, M.D., and Edmund R. Novak, M.D., eds. *Textbook of Gynecology.* Baltimore: Williams and Wilkins Co., 1956.

The next morning Sims attended a white woman who had been thrown from a horse and had landed on her pelvis. Remembering an early lesson from a teacher in medical school, Sims believed that he needed to "relocate" the uterus, an idea consistent with nineteenth-century medical beliefs that the uterus could easily dislodge from its proper place, causing untold emotional and physical problems. In order to "relocate" the uterus, he had the woman assume a position on her knees and elbows, covered her with a large sheet, inserted two fingers into her vagina, and found, just as his teacher had promised, that a suction was created that extended the vagina to full capacity.[24] This event caused Sims to reconsider his ability to repair fistulas. If the vagina would "puff up" in this position, then why couldn't he introduce an instrument that would enable him to visualize the fistula and thus repair it?

Conveniently enough, Lucy was still in Sims's backyard hospital. He bought a pewter spoon on his way home. Upon arrival, he hurriedly assembled his two medical student-apprentices and placed Lucy in the knee-chest position for examination: "Introducing the bent handle of the spoon I saw everything, as no man had ever seen before. The fistula was as plain as the nose on a man's face."[25] This historic moment has since achieved mythological status as the first use of a vaginal speculum, commonly known as Sims's speculum, in North America (see Figure 1).

"As plain as the nose on a man's face" is a strange expression to use in conjunction with the initial "discovery" of vaginal visibility. It is as though Sims saw his own image, a self-portrait, reflected back at him in the pewter spoon. I will consider the implications of the speculum as a place for self-reflection later in this chapter. What is significant is the fact that the speculum was "discovered" in a slave woman's body. Visibility, ownership, labor, capital, medical discovery, and slavery all met at the site of the first speculum exam.

The Speculum

Although vaginal speculums in various forms have been noted as early as A.D. 97, they had not found their way into modern American medical practice until Sims examined Lucy.[26] There is no question that the speculum is a highly significant technology and its discovery in part accounts for Sims's title, Father of Modern Gynecology. In eulogizing Sims, W. O. Baldwin, M.D., emphasized the instrument's importance: "The day which made him great was the day the idea of his speculum first dawned upon him—that day when he first conceived the thought of throwing an abundance of light into the vagina and around the womb, and at the same time obtaining ample space to work and ply his instruments. . . . The instrument caused his name to flash over the medical world like a meteor in the night. Gynaecology to-day would not deserve the name of a separate and cultivated science, but for the light which Sims's speculum and the principles involved in it have thrown upon it."[27]

Images of light and enlightenment abound in Baldwin's text. By "throwing an abundance of light" into the dark cavity, Sims made the invisible visible. One cannot help but recall here Freud's notion of woman as "the dark continent" and its "link to the nineteenth-century colonialist imagination."[28] If woman is dark, in this case doubly "dark" due to her mysterious anatomy and African origins, Sims is the source of enlightenment, constructing knowledge about her internal depths. In her discussion of medical stories in women's films of the 1940s, Mary Ann Doane has analyzed the continual narrative return to images of light. She notes, "Light also enables the look, the male gaze—it makes the woman specularizable. The doctor's light legitimates scopophilia."[29] The light introduced by Sims's speculum allowed for an entirely new medical specialty premised on the vaginal spectacle. Sims drew the labial curtains, propped open the vaginal walls, and revealed an entirely new vision; this accounts for his epithet: Architect of the Vagina. Making the internal structures of the live woman visible with the speculum allowed the enlightened knowledge of medical science to enter; physicians could now see and, therefore, manipulate this previously invisible zone. In this respect, the creation of the speculum participated in a Western medical tradition that was founded on visibility.[30] As in Luce Irigaray's notion of the speculum, the light thrown into the dark space is then reflected back onto the prestigious image of Sims himself, whose name flashed "over the medical world like a meteor in the night." Illuminating the inside of the vagina lit up his own career in the process, making him a guiding light to those physicians who had previously labored in the dark.

Baldwin, Sims's eulogizer, proceeds to compare the speculum to other great inventions: "It has been to diseases of the womb what the printing press is to civilization, what the compass is to the mariner, what steam is to navigation, what the telescope is to astronomy, and grander than the telescope because it was the work of one man."[31] In Baldwin's account, Sims alone discovered the instrument that would help organize the uncharted female landscape. This man-made invention was construed as yet another example of science's triumph over nature. The speculum served as yet another instance of man's progress in that it made visible the inner recesses of the female body, just as the telescope enabled a view of the outer depths of space. The speculum was like a compass in that it helped guide the physician into this unknown terrain. In this rhetorical construction, the female body is metaphorically produced as raw natural territory awaiting discovery and cultivation by the hands of male medical culture. On first using the speculum and viewing the inside of the vagina, Sims himself wrote: "I felt like an explorer in medicine who first views a new and important territory."[32] Without science the female body was unruly and nonsensical; the speculum helped organize and establish the female body, particularly the female reproductive organs, as a place suitable for, and open to, medical intervention.

The narrative formulas used to describe Sims's medical adventures present classic scenarios: a hero triumphantly overcoming trial and tribulation, fighting battles in order to conquer new lands, build new spaces, and create new orders.[33] Under all of this lies the female body, serving at once as obstacle and as object in need of discovery, conquering, and restructuring. Thus in historic writings about Sims, the female body, particularly the black female body, becomes what Teresa de Lauretis refers to as a "plot-space," marking the landscape through which Sims, the medical hero, traverses in order to find fame, knowledge, and wealth.[34]

Bearing the Pain

After Sims's first use of the pewter spoon and his view of "what no man had seen before," he asked Lucy to stay and requested that Anarcha and Betsey be sent back to him. Believing he was "on the eve of a great discovery," he asked their masters for consent: "I agree to perform no experiment or operation . . . to endanger their lives and will not charge a cent for keeping them, but you must pay their taxes and clothe them. I will keep them at my own expense."[35] Since Sims had already argued that these women could not properly perform their duties as servants due to their "disgusting condition," his offer must have seemed a good deal to the owners. He would not deplete their slave capital, but would sustain their lives himself and might even repair them and thus return them to their original value. The backyard hospital for slaves was enlarged, and Sims set about inventing instruments, setting the stage for a show that would be extended time and time again, finally closing after a four-year run.

Who were the slave women on whom Sims experimented? We know them from Sims's autobiography and subsequent biographical writings only by their first names. Did they have husbands, partners, children, and loved ones whom they were made to leave for four years while Sims worked on them? Did they agree to his experimentation? Were they given any choices? under what terms? What were their feelings toward their condition? Did they ever leave Sims's backyard hospital over the course of their tenure there? It is impossible to know. They did not write their own histories. Thus the ways in which Sims's surgeries related to these women's lives is left unknown; the documentation of their performances is subject to surviving writings mainly unconcerned with such incidental facts.

Lucy was the first to undergo surgery to suture together the edges of the fistula. With a patronizing flourish, Sims remarked on her fortitude: "That was before the days of anesthetics, and the poor girl, on her knees, bore the operation with great heroism and bravery."[36] The pain these women must have experienced during and following these operations is inconceivable. And as if the pain of unanesthetized vaginal surgery were not traumatic enough, after this first operation, Lucy nearly died from infection due to a sponge Sims had left in her urethra and bladder.

Sims and Harris depict the slave women as inherently more durable than white women. About one hundred years following the surgeries, Harris echoes Sims's racist patronizing: "Sims's experiments brought them physical pain, it is true, but they bore it with amazing patience and fortitude—a grim stoicism which may have been part of their racial endowment or which possibly had been bred into them through several generations of enforced submission."[37] Causing the slave women great pain did not deter Sims from proceeding with the operations. Not only were the painful punishments administered to slave women by masters and overseers seen as a kind of "preparation" for the rigors of unanesthetized surgery, but slaves were viewed as genetically more predisposed than whites to the kind of domestication that trained them to bear pain.[38]

Pathologizing Difference

Other cultural and historical factors allowed Sims to believe that slave women were appropriate subjects for such painful experimentation. It was possible for

Sims to operate repeatedly and unabashedly on slave women subjects in part because these women were viewed as abundantly symptomatic and pathological. Given a cultural backdrop that pathologized race and black female sexuality alike, slave women with vesico-vaginal fistulas were triply symptomatic. Their first pathological symptom was their primary racial characteristic: their skin color. In a medical world that categorized life as either normal or pathological, people of the African diaspora were continually condemned to the category of pathological, their "abnormal" skin color serving as a foil for "normal" white skin. Pathological causes for this condition were concocted in order to explain its prevalence. Sander Gilman explains: "Medical tradition has a long history of perceiving this skin color as the result of some pathology. The favorite theory, which reappears with some frequency in the early nineteenth century, is that skin color and attendant physiognomy of the black are the result of congenital leprosy."[39] Such medical arguments, in collusion with racist and stereotypic scientific and cultural explanations and excuses, provided the grounds for differential "treatment."

The slave woman's second symptom was her sex, taken in combination with her skin color. Black female sexuality and sex characteristics were the site of great attention by a nineteenth-century scientific community that systematically found them to be pathological.[40] Black female sexuality, constructed as heathen, lascivious, and excessive, was used by dominant nineteenth-century scientific culture to counter its constructions of fragile and frigid (and also pathological) white female sexuality.[41] These differing constructions of white and black female sexualities may account for the fact that Mrs. Merrill, the white woman who had been thrown from a horse, was covered with a sheet during examination, whereas unanesthetized Lucy underwent Sims's first experimental surgery while "about a dozen" male spectators watched. The spectacle of Lucy's genital display did not require limiting the number of spectators or providing an obscuring sheet. In this way, slave women may have been seen as more appropriate objects of study, for the experimenting physician believed that he need not worry about protecting the slave's modesty.

In the early nineteenth century, white European researchers documented physical evidence to provide proof of pathology. Black female genitals and "steatopygia" (protruding buttocks) were singled out as telling sites of difference and pathology. In their trips to Africa, researchers commented on the "primitive" genitalia of African women, particularly Bushman and Hottentot. Named the "Hottentot Venus," Saartje Baartman (also referred to as Sarah Bartmann) was exhibited in Europe for over five years. She was clothed during live exhibition so her buttocks were of greater interest than the hidden genitalia. But following her death in 1815 in Paris, her genitalia took the spotlight: "The audience that had paid to see Sarah Bartmann's buttocks and fantasized about her genitalia could, after her death and dissection, examine both."[42] Following her death, George Cuvier, a pathologist, presented "the Academy the genital organs of this woman prepared in a way so as to allow one to see the nature of the labia."[43] The postmortem museum display of the Hottentot Venus's genitalia is reminiscent of Barnum's orchestration of Joice Heth's theatricalized autopsy. The surgical theater and museum display, spaces often reserved for serious scientific investigation, become Barnum sideshows. In both cases, public display of what is normally private—the genitals or the inside of the body—was used as evidence of freakish abnormalities. The genitalia of the Hottentot woman became the marker of her inherent pathology, her sex parts serving as a metonym for her pathological sexuality and therefore as fitting representatives for inclusion in an anatomical museum.

Given this historical context of the continual pathologizing of black women, the third pathological symptom and only legitimate abnormality, the vesicovaginal fistula, made these slave women ideal subjects for study. The vesicovaginal tears, located in the mysterious inner cavity, were only accessible by a physician's probing fingers and tools. There were persistent questions regarding the moral and ethical appropriateness of examining white women's genitals and reproductive organs; Western society questioned the suitability of a physician penetrating such a private place traditionally reserved for the patient's husband.[44] Yet with the slave, these questions were laid to rest. She was not only white man's property, but because of her racially legitimized pathological "nature," she was considered promiscuous and sexually voracious. The need to manipulate the slave's genitals in search of the vesico-vaginal fistula made her an apt surgical recipient.

Utilizing Sameness

Difference was vital to Sims's experiments. The slave's triple pathology allowed him to perform multiple operations. Western medical and scientific men in the nineteenth century tried to prove black female difference, as is evidenced in the actual display of Sarah Bartmann's external genitals. Yet Sims's experiments were also premised on an internal sameness, his invention of the speculum providing the tool that allowed such sameness to be examined. If he could successfully mend a slave woman's fistula, then it was assumed that he would be able to repair *any* woman's fistula. This simultaneous sameness and difference is what made the slave women such fitting "human guinea pigs."[45] Slavery provided the ideal conditions for Sims's surgical experimentation. As we have seen, convenient racial pathologies legitimated surgical manipulation and unabashed pelvic observation of the slave women, while their palpably (and now visibly) analogous insides made them suitable white female correlates.

In Baldwin's eulogizing of Sims, he proclaims, "The time was ripe when Sims patiently began to work out problems which were essential to operative gynaecology. Even slavery had its uses in the pursuit of his ends. Who can tell how many more years the progress of the art might have been delayed if the humble Negro servitors had not brought their willing sufferings and patient endurance to aid in the furthering of Sims's purpose."[46] "The time was ripe" indeed, but not necessarily for the reasons that Baldwin asserts. Who was actually offering the slaves' "willing sufferings . . . to aid in the furthering of Sims's purpose"? Of course, it was the slave owners rather than the slaves themselves who initiated contact with Sims and who had the final say as to whether their slaves could remain in Sims's care. "The time was ripe" because Sims, an already reputable body mechanic, offered these masters a promising proposition: he would repair their laborer, making her fit for her duties. In a slave economy, this surgery held particular value. Not only did it repair the slave capital so she could work, but by ridding her of the fistula's "loathsome" and "disgusting" attributes the surgery also affected her likelihood to reproduce, a vital aspect of her role as slave.

Harris suggests that there were even greater risks to having a fistula. He maintains that some slave women were led to suicide by their "loathsome" condition. Harris's statement suggests that Sims's experimentation was really for the slave women's benefit. However, we may further ask, as Diana Axelsen has in an essay on Sims, how severe a disorder a vesico-vaginal fistula truly is and whether it merited such extreme attention: "While certainly a source of chronic discomfort and possible secondary irritation, and while obviously embarrassing in many contexts, vesico-vaginal fistula is not a disorder involving chronic or severe pain . . . the discomfort of vesico-vaginal fistula, in comparison to the effects of excessive beatings, chronic malnutrition, and other forms of physical and psychological aggression, hardly constitutes a probable motive for suicide."[47] Not to mention the tremendous agony of unanesthetized vaginal surgery. The pain and suffering these women endured was hardly a break from hardship. While none of the women undergoing Sims's experimentation committed suicide, four years of unanesthetized surgery on one's vagina might have been a much more likely motive than the vesico-vaginal fistula itself.

Lucy did not die following Sims's first surgical attempt but survived the infection, healing in due course for her subsequent operations. More slaves came to live in Sims's backyard: "Besides these three cases, I got three or four more to experiment on, and there was never a time that I could not, at any day, have had a subject for operation."[48] Sims rotated operations on his slave patients, but could not make the operation work. Each time he would make adjustments to the procedure, but there was always a small fistula remaining, and a small fistula had the same result as a large fistula: it leaked. As one patient was healing, he would operate on the next (who would have just finished healing from her last operation), incorporating his latest surgical innovation.

Those physicians and students who had initially attended the operations, eagerly awaiting Sims's great success, lost interest. Without assistants, he trained the slave women to assist in each other's operations.[49] Thus the slave's role shifted throughout the surgical process: slave as laboring assistant or stage hand, slave as repairable capital, and slave as medical guinea pig. Women, particularly women of color, have been cast most often in similar roles throughout Western medical history: as either nurse, technician, or nonphysician assistant, and as subject of experimentation and manipulation particularly with regard to reproductive organs.[50] Their power in the medical apparatus has reflected the roles they have been assigned. However, since the abolition of slavery, the nature of the experimentation and manipulation of African American women's reproductivity has shifted with the changing status of African American women as reproductive capital.

Three years after Sims's experiments began, his brother-in-law, Dr. Rush Jones, visited Sims and implored him to discontinue his work on the slaves. He told Sims that he was working too much, that the cost of supporting the slaves was high, and that he was being unfair to his family. According to Sims's and Harris's accounts, Jones did not raise concerns about the slaves' welfare. However, Harris does note that there was talk in the community: "And socially the whole business was becoming a marked liability, for all kinds of whispers were beginning to circulate around town—dark rumors that it was a terrible thing for Sims to be allowed to keep on using human beings as experimental animals for his unproven surgical theories."[51] Nowhere else in Sims's biography or autobiography is there mention of the possible ways in which his treatment of the slaves was unethical. Rather, it is continuously emphasized that the slaves were there out of desperation and in the hope that Sims might rid them of their condition. In response to the townspeople's uneasiness with Sims's practice, Harris emphasizes that "the human guinea pigs themselves, however, made no complaints on this score." He uses the term "human guinea pigs" ironically here to imply the slave women's willing acceptance of their role as experimental animal, even though "dark rumors" were being spread around town. However, in an article on Sims in *Journal of Medical Ethics*, Durrenda Ojanuga asserts that the women "were in no way volunteers for Dr. Sims's research." In fact, "the evidence suggests that Sims's use of slave women as experimental subjects was by no means the order of the day!"[52] Thus Sims's practices cannot be viewed as historically acceptable or commonplace. Yet it is important to remember that these practices, nonetheless, instituted the foundation of gynecology as a distinct specialty.

Sims's tenacity in battling the fistula despite criticism from his relatives, friends, and colleagues is highlighted by both Sims and his biographer. He is rhetorically placed on a research team with the slaves in a dedicated search for a cure for their ailments. In the writings, it is as though no power differential existed between Sims and his experimentees. But the slaves themselves would not become famous; it was Sims who would wear the honors. According to Harris, Sims was so driven that when Jones begged him to stop the experimentation, Sims was steadfast in his commitment. As Harris describes: "It was like advising a dog that he will be out of breath if he doesn't stop chasing a squirrel—like advising Columbus to turn back because the voyage is long and there is no land in sight. Sims, once aroused, was a zealot."[53] Even eighty years later the characterization of the slave woman as "dark continent" had not died out. Metaphors similar to the ones used to remark on Sims's speculum in 1883 were used by Harris to remark on Sims's actions. Once again, the slave body is metaphorized as an unruly, uncharted, dark continent containing rich mysteries and spicy secrets. While the explorer utilizes the telescope or compass, the physician dealing in female disorders will make use of the speculum. Sims, like Columbus, was determined to conquer a naturalized resource (the Americas or the female body), civilizing the previously "uncivilized" territory. Fame was at stake for both, dependent on brutality, racist notions of entitlement, and the institution of slavery. However, less glamorous than the comparison to Columbus, Sims is also referred to as a dog chasing the wild squirrel of surgical success. With the Columbus and dog metaphors, ideas of driven and instinctual behavior, exploration, conquest, and domestication are joined as a means of legitimizing racial and sexual domination.

Throughout his experiments, Sims made adjustments in the hopes of successful surgery. Each time he was frustrated by the small fistula that remained. Deciding he needed a different type of suture, he traded in his silk thread for a silver wire suture that he had had specially made, and the fistula was repaired. He considered his silver sutures to be "the greatest surgical achievement of the nineteenth century."[54] In the summer of 1849 he operated on Anarcha, the first fistula case he had ever seen, and the operation was a success. It was Anarcha's thirtieth operation.

Master Showman's Second Act

In 1855 Sims founded the Woman's Hospital in New York, a place where women could go despite their economic circumstances. The hospital was the first ever dedicated to female disorders and its wards were largely filled with destitute Irish immigrant women.[55] It would appear that this was a charity hospital for the good of the poor. But as was the case with the slaves in Sims's backyard, patients at the Woman's Hospital were frequently kept there "indefinitely" and underwent multiple surgeries. From 1856 to 1859, an early indigent Irish visitor to the Woman's Hospital, Mary Smith, survived thirty operations, the same number Anarcha endured in Sims's backyard. However, it must not be forgotten that these women, unlike the slaves, had the benefits of anesthetics. Before Sims was aware of the existence of anesthestics he had attempted surgery on white women, "but they seemed unable to bear the operation's pain and discomfort with the stoicism shown by the Negroes."[56] However, the widespread use of anesthestics finally allowed Sims to bring his surgeries to white women and allowed for the establishment of places such as the Woman's Hospital. The Woman's Hospital continually provided Sims with bodies on which he could experiment with new surgeries and instruments. Discoveries he made at the hospital were then utilized in his private practice in exchange for high fees.[57]

Sims moved to Europe during the Civil War, retaining his position as a "loyal southerner."[58] With the help of anesthestics, Sims operated on numerous wealthy European women, including a countess in France; he often had large audiences filling his operating theater to capacity. He stayed in Paris, where he was a "hit": "Here I performed in the amphitheatre, in which Joubard de Lamballe had performed all his operations."[59] Thus he clearly measured his success by the surgeon stars who had frequented the same stage.

When Sims returned to New York with his European fame and confidence, he took center stage, making the Woman's Hospital into his own private experimentation theater—scores of medical men came to observe Sims's performance of daring surgeries. Here he performed controversial surgeries as well, including Battey's operation, which Sims helped "make respectable." In the 1870s Battey's operation, or bilateral ovariotomy (removal of both ovaries), became a fashionable surgery to "treat" a variety of illnesses including insanity, epilepsy, and nervous disorders that were believed to originate in the female reproductive organs.[60] The operation had the added effect of sterilization.

On his return from Europe with his new titles, Knight Commander of the Legion of Honor of France, Knight of the Order of Isabella the Catholic of Spain, and Knight of the Order of Leopold I of Belgium, there was new concern about Sims's practices. His biographer attributes this to his contemporaries' jealousy of and weariness over Sims's success: "He was too cocksure, they felt, too reckless, too much inclined to hold the spotlight in a one-man starring part." The

Board of Lady Managers, a group of rich white women who oversaw the "moral and domestic management" of the Woman's Hospital and whose help Sims himself had solicited in order to afford his hospital legitimacy, recognized that Sims was experimenting on his patients and objected to the large audiences Sims allowed into his operating theater. A Lady Managers' memorandum asks, "Is the Woman's Hospital to be made a public school or is it to be a Private Hospital where our afflicted Sisters can come without fear?"[61] They limited to fifteen the number of spectators allowed during operations. Outraged, Sims resigned from the hospital in 1875 and a few months later was elected president of the AMA, his well-publicized resignation apparently rewarded by this esteemed organization. In his presidential address he attacked the AMA's code of ethics which oversees and disciplines physicians' practices. Sims asked his colleagues, "Did it ever occur to you that [the AMA's code of ethics] is capable of being used as an engine of torture and oppression?" Sims felt that the code was too strict, as reflected by the medical establishment's unease with some of Sims's practices.[62]

Throughout the latter part of his career Sims invented new tools and techniques for "treating" women. Contemporaneous with sterilizing the mentally disordered, Sims was seeking out innovative solutions to correct private patients' infertility. For example, he invented and used an instrument for the amputation of the cervix which he called the "uterine guillotine." A pioneer in artificial insemination, Sims was also taken with the practice of "splitting the cervix" supposedly in order to ease the travel of semen and menses through the cervical canal. Many gynecologists considered the practice "butcherous."[63] Coining the term "vaginismus" to refer to female "frigidity," a condition that disallows penetration by the penis into the vagina, Sims proceeded to invent a number of methods to remedy the situation, including hymenotomy (the operation discussed in the previous chapter), incising the vaginal orifice, and dilating the vagina with various-sized wedges. In "treating" vaginismus, Sims would sometimes simply anesthetize the woman so that her husband could have intercourse with her in order to impregnate her. This procedure asserted the compatibility of the passive, anesthetized female body with gynecological as well as sexual manipulation. In the following chapter, we will see this relationship mirrored one hundred years later in the use of anesthetized women for teaching medical students how to perform pelvic exams. The passive, powerless female pelvis is thus situated as a model receptacle for medical intervention.

Sims continued to enlist such passive female bodies in order to prove his master showmanship. In 1879, four years prior to his death, Sims threw a gala event, something between a trade show and a circus. For four days, he performed a series of varied operations on different women, ending in a dinner at Sims's house for fifty or sixty physicians.[64] As if in response to the Board of Lady Managers' reprimand of Sims for his large audiences at the Woman's Hospital, the gala event openly defied the Lady Managers' protocol for proper surgical performance.

Between Sims and the Board of Lady Managers, the staging of the operative performance had been called into question. The Lady Managers disputed Sims's previously unlimited power over the type of gaze and manipulation practiced on his patients' bodies. But the gaze he wished to have control over was not only his own, but that of his audience-followers. Throughout his medical career, Sims was always in the spotlight; after Sims enlisted anesthestics, his patients were even more proplike than before. The fact that the patients at the Woman's Hospital were white undoubtedly influenced the Lady Managers' idea of appropriate modesty. Because of their race and position within antebellum southern society, the slave women had been more appropriate objects for exhibition.

The appropriateness of the slave women for exhibition and unanesthetized experimentation served as a legitimation of the institution of slavery, as is evident in Sims's eulogist's statement that "the time was ripe" for Sims's experimentation. Implicit in this statement is the idea that the ends, gynecology and the furtherance of medicine, justified the means, slavery. The implication is that it is fortunate for humanity in general that slavery existed if only because it helped foster medical innovation. And as we can see from Sims's practices following slavery, his attitudes toward women, their bodies, and reproductivity were undoubtedly affected by his long-time experimentation on slave women. Gynecology in the United States evolved through the bodies of slave women. While slavery was eventually abolished, inequality and institutionalized racism flourishes. Certain populations, particularly poor women of color, are still viewed as more fitting experimentees for, and more fitting recipients of, new technologies than other populations. Unfortunately, the time is still ripe and medical innovation is still the excuse.

Sims continues to be praised in the introductions to gynecology texts and medical history books without reference to his questionable practices. When his practices are questioned, as they were in a 1970s article that appeared in the *American Journal of Obstetrics and Gynecology* titled "Reappraisals of James Marion Sims," many physicians were outraged and defended Sims. The author, Irwin H. Kaiser, M.D., was not particularly critical of Sims and even responded to Barker-Benfield's chapter on Sims in *Horrors of the Half-Known Life* that although "Sims was insensitive to the status and needs of women," he was simply a "product of his era," and that one must "be skeptical of judging 1850 decisions by 1975 norms." Kaiser's colleagues, as evidenced by their discussions following his piece, were outraged by *any* questioning of Sims's practices. Dr. Denis Cavanagh responded, "Lest this distinguished Society degenerate into just another social club, we all have a responsibility to supply the program committee with good scientific papers. In my opinion this paper damns Sims with faint praise and is one of the least impressive papers that I have heard before this society." Dr. Lawrence L. Hester Jr. concurred: "I rise not to reappraise J. Marion Sims, but to praise him—to praise him as the father of gynecology and not to condemn him as an exploiter of women." These responses illustrate the vehemence with which Sims's work has been supported.[65]

While such a staunch defense of Sims might not commonly be found in print twenty years later, it is as significant that the evolution of the specialty of gynecology is not openly considered and questioned in medical texts and medical history books. If gynecology is premised on such practices, might the entire specialty be reconsidered in this light? If it were, we would surely find that the racism and misogyny underlying Sims's practices still flourish in contemporary medicine and its applications, particularly with regard to women and their reproductive organs. The decisions made in the mid-nineteenth century continue to directly and indirectly influence the lives of women today. This does not mean that practitioners have studied Sims or are aware of his historic importance. Rather the medical apparatus continues to accommodate and even reward such racism and misogyny.

Sims's experiments on slave women, his practice of ovariotomy on the mentally disabled, and his pioneering work in artificial insemination and infertility helped institute the idea that it was appropriate for medical professionals to seek out new ways of both limiting and fostering female reproductivity. Forever in search of a new tool or surgical technique, Sims was one of the earliest physicians to link female reproductivity with a kind of technophilia, publishing extensively on each new innovation. Sims's work also linked experimentation on the female reproductive organs to race and power, since his earliest experiments were executed on female slaves.

In order to explore the legacy of Sims's work, I will consider the contraceptive technology Norplant. Experiments with Norplant were conducted almost exclusively on poor third world women, and since its FDA approval in 1990 it has been coercively and even legislatively aimed at poor women of color in the United States and abroad as a solution to the threat of their reproductivity. Whereas new technologies that limit reproductivity are often aimed at poor women of color, concurrently new reproductive technologies that extend or promote fertility (e.g., in vitro fertilization) are largely aimed at wealthy, white women. The impetus to enhance or contain reproductivity on the basis of race or social status can be traced to Sims's early practices.

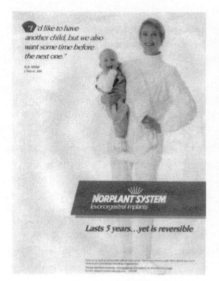
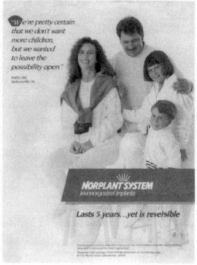

Whereas Sims's vesico-vaginal fistula operations can be viewed as one of the earliest reproductive technologies, enhancing slaves' reproductive capacities and thus allowing them to continue their "duties" as "breeders," Norplant is a form of temporary sterilization that prevents reproductivity. The historical conditions out of which each technology arose explain their opposite aims. Sims conducted his experiments at a time when the ruling southern whites could benefit from the reproductivity of slave women; Norplant has been developed as a response to the alleged need for new ways of controlling poor women's reproductivity given the rhetorical backdrop of welfare crises and overpopulation. While arising out of very different historical conditions, Norplant and Sims's crude reproductive technologies are cousins. Both in Sims's time and today, certain women's reproductivity is valued over others', and new technologies are demanded in order to foster and prevent reproduction.

"Welcome to a New Era in Contraceptive Technology"[66]

Approved by the FDA in 1990, Norplant is a subdermal contraceptive consisting of six small silicone rubber capsules that are surgically implanted in a woman's arm. The capsules diffuse a synthetic progesterone, levonorgestrel, that effectively inhibits ovulation and thickens cervical mucous, preventing pregnancy for up to five years. Because it is surgically implanted and removed, Norplant is

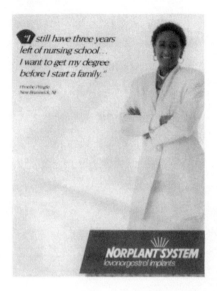

"I still have three years left of nursing school... I want to get my degree before I start a family."

Phoebe Pringle
New Brunswick, NJ

NORPLANT SYSTEM
levonorgestrel implants

Figure 2. Norplant advertisement.
In *The Nurse Practitioner* (May 1992).
Figure 3. Norplant advertisement.
In *The Nurse Practitioner* (June 1992).
Figure 4. Norplant advertisement.
In *The Nurse Practitioner* (May 1989).

physician controlled and "user soft." Theoretically, the user cannot designate when to start and stop Norplant; rather a health practitioner must insert and remove the capsules, making Norplant particularly prone to institutional abuse. Norplant has been especially attractive to the international population control industry, for whom technologies that are effective, low maintenance, and provider dependent are valued. Norplant is mainly used in developing countries in Asia, Latin America, and Africa. The majority of Norplant's clinical or preintroduction studies were conducted in developing countries as well. Some fifty-five thousand women were included in these studies.[67]

This seemingly science fictive technology confirms the medical industry's presumption, asserted if not established by Sims, of the compatibility of the female body, particularly the female reproductive organs, with new technologies. Norplant, yet another case of science triumphing over nature, has been heralded throughout the world as a panacea technology. From Egypt, where the national press referred to Norplant as "the magic capsule," to the United States, where it has been heralded as "a birth control breakthrough," Norplant has received praise for its remarkable possibilities.

Its high-tech appeal was taken up by Norplant's advertising agents when they constructed a series of ads that pictured women meeting the viewer's gaze while responding to the question "Why do you choose Norplant?" White woman and white family are dressed in white on a white background, constructing users as overwhelmingly modern, wealthy, and white (see Figures 2 and 3). Often, a con-

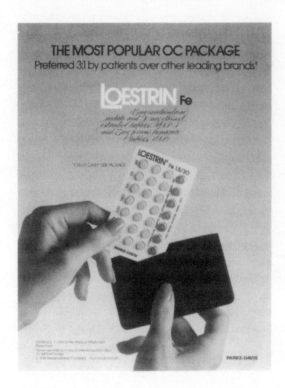

Figure 5. Loestrin
advertisement. In *The Nurse
Practitioner* (July 1992).

traceptive is at the center of the frame in pharmaceutical advertising (see Figure 5); that is, the product itself is pictured. However, because Norplant is placed within the body, it is absent from the image, indicating that the woman shown has already securely incorporated Norplant into her modern body. One ad does picture an African American woman (see Figure 3). She too is dressed in the uniform white and set against a white background. Her reasons for choosing Norplant are not those of her white counterparts, who have either temporarily reached optimal family size or are taking a break between children. Rather, the woman represented wishes to finish school; she wishes to enter into a viable socioeconomic space that would allow her to support her future baby. Issues of supporting the young white children pictured in the ads previously shown are left unaddressed. It is assumed that personal, not economically motivated choice is the reason a white woman or white family would decide to stop reproducing. The single African American woman, pictured childless, is given an economic reason and a societally acceptable one at that.

Both technological innovations, Norplant and Sims's vesico-vaginal surgeries, are proposed as ways of helping black women be more "fit for their duties."

Sims's vesico-vaginal fistula reparations would make the slave women more fit for their duties as breeders. In a slave economy, it is economically beneficial to those in power to repair slave capital so that she and her future progeny may provide labor. The slave woman's reproductivity must be reclaimed *from* pathology. In a capitalist welfare economy, the reproductivity of poor women of color *is* her pathology. In the former case, reproductivity is economically beneficial to those with capital; in the latter reproductivity is believed to deplete economic resources. Whereas the slave women Sims experimented on were attributed a triple dose of pathology—race, sex, fistula—poor women of color today are still pathologized for the first two (race and sex), but reproductivity replaces the fistula as the third pathology.

Slave masters encouraged adolescent slave girls to have children;[68] now "teenage pregnancy," predominantly associated with poor women of color, is linked with gangs and drugs as an evil of modern society. Norplant is seen as a new technology that can help put an end to teenage pregnancy and restore racial "balance" to the U.S. population. In December 1992, the front page of the *New York Times* told the story well. An article with the headline "Population Growth Outstrips Earlier U.S. Census Estimates" showed projections into the year 2050, where "white" population growth would remain steady while black, Asian, and Hispanic populations would double at the very least.[69] Bedfellows with this front-page article was another piece titled "Baltimore School Clinics to Offer Birth Control by Surgical Implant."[70] It is no surprise that the large majority of young women affected by this decision in the Baltimore area are poor African Americans. Norplant will not protect these teens from sexually transmitted diseases or educate them about their bodies and pregnancy, nor had any medical research addressed the health risks of Norplant in women under the age of twenty at the time such decisions were made. Norplant is used as a "quick fix" to the high teen birthrate in the Baltimore area and as a means of remedying uneven population growth.

Poor African American women who do have many children, women that ex-Senator Russell B. Long referred to as "Black Brood Mares,"[71] are often disdained for leeching tax dollars. The duties of African American women today are viewed by the dominant culture as opposite to those of her slave ancestors. No longer is the African American woman in the Norplant ad expected to breed for her oppressors; now, new technologies such as Norplant aid her in becoming an educated, income-earning member of society *before* she has children. The narrative of these ads suggests that Norplant in fact serves a purpose similar to Sims's reparative surgeries, playing into current dominant constructions of proper African American women's reproductive identity.

If poor women, particularly poor African American women, are not "fit for their duties," securing proper earning potential before they have children, Norplant has been seen as a technology that can remedy such misbehavior. The *Philadelphia Inquirer* published an editorial two days following FDA approval in December 1990, suggesting readers think about using Norplant as a "tool in the fight against African-American poverty."[72] A few weeks later, California judge Howard Broadman ordered Darlene Johnson, a twenty-seven-year-old pregnant African American mother of four who had been convicted of child abuse, to have Norplant inserted or to serve a jail sentence.[73] In 1993 Washington State, Arizona, Colorado, Ohio, Tennessee, North Carolina, South Carolina, and Florida all proposed incentive-based or mandate-based welfare reform linked to Norplant. For example, the proposal in Ohio would increase monthly Aid to Families with Dependent Children (AFDC) payments and offer a $500 incentive for Norplant insertion or $1000 for sterilization. If a woman chose not to use Norplant and subsequently became pregnant, her benefits might be discontinued entirely or they might not be increased with the birth of the child. In Florida, the proposed reform set AFDC benefits at $258 per month regardless of the number of children in the family, but a recipient with an effective implant would receive $400 per month.[74] As the National Black Women's Health Project's newsletter asserts, "the line between incentive and coercion is fuzzy. The incentives are only being offered for one contraceptive—Norplant—to one class of women—poor, single, mothers on welfare—who are more likely women of color—what happened to choice?"[75]

Women on welfare receive incentives for temporary or permanent sterilization; slave women received incentives such as better rations for prolific reproduction. It is unclear, however, what the slaves' "incentives" were for submitting to Sims's repeated surgeries. In their writings, Sims and Harris altogether disavow questions of the slaves' choice or consent by maintaining that the slave women were eager to be cured, willingly submitted to surgery, and even participated in the surgeries as Sims's assistants. Their positions as slaves authorized their "willingness" and consent, as they already had few legitimate choices regarding their bodies and everyday activities.[76] Similarly, we might consider how much "choice" a poor woman on welfare has when faced with such options regarding Norplant. And this "choice" is not as clear-cut as it may seem. Norplant does not serve as a simple on-and-off switch for fertility: there are a host of side effects that may accompany its use. The most common is a change in menstrual bleeding patterns. A significant number of women will bleed on and off throughout their cycle for the first year of use.[77] Other side effects include dizziness, headaches, nervousness, weight gain, weight loss, ovarian cysts, acne, infections at the implant site, nipple discharge, inflammation of the cervix, mood changes, depression, general malaise, itching, and hypertension.[78] The term "side effect" belittles the crushing impact any one of these symptoms may have on an individual's life.

Despite these foreboding possibilities, internal Population Council documents show that women in Indonesia, Bangladesh, and numerous other countries had difficulties getting Norplant removed due to resistant trial investigators whose scientific data "would be rendered incomplete."[79] Likewise, in early clinical trials done with Norplant, many cases of abuse regarding informed consent have been noted in numerous countries, including Indonesia, Brazil, Thailand, and Egypt. Medical innovation and experimentation are again used to legitimate oppression and control over the bodies of poor women of color. As in the case of Sims's experiments, it is "difference"—in this case, poor women of color's pathological race, sexuality, and reproductivity—that legitimates Norplant experiments and the product's continued use. And yet such studies are premised on a convenient user "sameness"—that Norplant will work identically on all female bodies, therefore women of color will be adequate testing grounds for technologies to be potentially used on higher-valued white bodies in the future, if they so choose. Balanced between Western pharmaceutical companies, the medical establishment, and assorted governmental bodies, one finds a distinct colonialist attitude at work, not dissimilar to the rhetoric underlying writings about Sims. Dominant white forces go to faraway lands to identify their sameness with the exotic "other," while simultaneously establishing and maintaining the other's difference and reaping the benefits of the new land and culture.

In many states in the United States a woman on public aid who has received free Norplant is in a position similar to that of third world women facing resistant trial investigators; she can only have Norplant removed if a practitioner deems it medically necessary.[80] Changes in menstrual bleeding patterns, the most common Norplant side effect, are not considered by the medical establishment to be a reason to discontinue its use. And yet this single side effect may deeply affect the cultural performance of some women, particularly Native American and Muslim women. A report on Norplant issued by the Native American Women's Health Education Resource Center reads: "for Native American women, the bleeding restricts their daily activity and prohibits them from participation in many traditional practices and religious ceremonies. . . . They do not attend sundances, sweats, or other spiritual ceremonies or go to any place where the pipe is used or to meetings of the Native American church. They also refrain from sexual activity. Ironically, the primary purpose of contraception— the ability to be sexually active without fear of pregnancy—then becomes a moot point."[81] Norplant users are from a variety of ethnic backgrounds and engage in a variety of cultural practices that are not factored into the statistical and biological studies conducted by the pharmaceutical and medical institutions. Such "difference" is not considered significant alongside the benefits of Norplant as an effective, ethnicity-blind technology for "controlling" populations.

"It's Your Choice"[82]

Temporary sterilization in the form of hormonal contraceptives is a common visitor to foreign lands. Norplant is not the first contraceptive to be tried on women of color in its early stages of development. Poor women of color in developing countries are used consistently as experimental subjects in order to test new hormonal contraceptive technologies before they are used on North American women.[83] The high-dose birth control pill and Depo-Provera, an injectable contraceptive, have each undergone these contraceptive trials, presenting women with a host of side effects and unknown long-lasting effects all under the auspices of population control.

Norplant, a form of temporary sterilization, is a participant in a form of eugenics deeply indebted to older, cruder technologies such as permanent sterilization. Norplant's newness and technological sophistication help mask its appropriation for the same racist patterns of behavior that resulted in the systematic coercive and abusive sterilization of huge numbers of women of color in Puerto Rico, the continental United States, and abroad beginning in the 1940s. By 1968, one-third of the women of childbearing age on the island of Puerto Rico had been sterilized. Most women sterilized had not been informed that the operation was, for all intents and purposes, irreversible.[84] Once again, one of the reasons these women were sterilized was so they could "fulfill their duties" as defined by U.S. manufacturing industries who needed cheap labor: "sterilization was perceived as a way to help 'free' them for employment, as opposed to, for example, providing good child-care facilities."[85]

Funds from the United States were often involved in sterilization campaigns. For example, in the early 1980s the World Bank Project funded a program in Bangladesh that would give starving women relief wheat if they would be sterilized. Women also received monetary awards and a sari and sarong. In addition, physicians and staff received incentives for each woman who agreed to sterilization.[86] At that time, the director of obstetrics and gynecology at a New York municipal hospital explained, "In most major teaching hospitals in New York City, it is the unwritten policy to do elective hysterectomies on poor black and Puerto Rican women, with minimal indications, to train residents."[87] Sterilization abuse has been widespread and disastrous, affecting the lives of many women who have had to live with choiceless futures.

In the United States, the most flagrant abuses took place between 1970 and 1976.[88] Alabama, the home of Sims's backyard hospital, was also the state in which, more than a century later, two black teenagers were sterilized without their consent or knowledge. This incident, known as the Relf case, was tried in the early 1970s; the court found "uncontroverted evidence in the record that minors and other incompetents have been sterilized with federal funds and that an indefinite number of poor people have been improperly coerced into accepting a sterilization operation under the threat that various federally supported welfare benefits would be withdrawn unless they submitted to irreversible sterilization."[89] The "incompetents" referred to here include mentally retarded and imprisoned women. These practices harken back to those of the Father of Modern Gynecology. As noted earlier, Sims himself practiced "female castration" on the "mentally disordered." Now such practices are taken up by Norplant. When introduced into Finland, its birthplace, Norplant was viewed as an inappropriate method for the majority of women but was targeted at very specific populations, one of them being "asocial women" (incarcerated, mentally ill, etc.). The category "asocial women" was "included in a commercial list of possible users given out by the manufacturer."[90] Though Norplant was viewed as an inappropriate method for most Finnish women, it was pushed as a first choice for many women of color. Certain women are deemed to be more fit users than others: As Purvis asks, "Are the women deemed 'unfit for motherhood' deemed fit for Norplant use?"[91] Whether subject to temporary or permanent sterilization or surgical reparation, the kinds of women targeted for medically sanctioned social control of their reproductivity—poor women, women of color, "asocial women"—are historically echoed.

Hidden Visibility

In the rhetoric surrounding Sims's practices, the importance of making visible the inner recesses of the female body is clear. It was necessary for Sims to invent the speculum so that he could visualize the vagina in order to ply his instruments. The speculum made Sims famous, his future practices dependent on such visibility. As a technology, Norplant displaces the vagina or pelvis as the site of intervention. Norplant is not about spectacular visual display. Rather it is about spectacular miniature technology, a modern means of mastering the female pelvis. It is heralded because it is hidden. In addition, practitioners do not have to "get their hands dirty" by viewing or manipulating the reproductive organs themselves. Norplant enlists a different theater of operations. The inner arm becomes a control booth for the reproductive organs from which the six silicone satellites release their hormones. Sims's daring and spectacular surgical feats are met today by technologies that regulate the female reproductive organs from afar.

Norplant's manufacturer's claims about its invisibility has come under fire. There is concern that Norplant, particularly in thin women, *does* mark the body. The capsules are indeed visible, serving as a sort of contraceptive tattoo or brand. The implications of these markings for population control are ominous.[92] In addition, scarring, particularly among women prone to keloids (African, African American, Middle Eastern, Mediterranean, etc.), has been a problem for many women using Norplant and one of the factors that led to a class action suit originating in Chicago on behalf of scarred users.[93] The women involved in this suit stated that they were not properly informed before insertion. Although Norplant's distributors claim that it may be surgically removed in twenty minutes, some users have had a string of removal attempts, resulting in broken capsules (with large amounts of hormones flooding the body), excruciating pain, and significant scarring.

Besides the many cases of inadequate preinsertion counseling and informed consent,[94] one of the worst problems associated with Norplant use abroad as well as in this country is the woman's difficulty having Norplant removed. Many women, particularly poor women, have trouble finding practitioners who will agree to its removal: either practitioners are trained in insertion and not removal or they do not deem the woman's removal request medically necessary.[95] Having control over when and how one has surgery is largely a factor of a woman's social status, thus directly related to race, class, and economics. This was as true in Sims's time as it is today. After Sims had operated twice on a white woman, Miss C., for a harelip, he "was eager to perfect his handiwork with a third" operation.[96] However, Miss C. refused, satisfied after two operations. The slaves in Sims's backyard hospital and the indigent women at the Woman's Hospital in New York did not have such clear options.

Nor do poor women today. In my work at a women's health clinic, I have heard stories—horrifying but not unexpected stories—of women so pained by Norplant's effects on their bodies and frustrated by the unwillingness of medical practitioners that they attempted to remove the implanted capsules from their own arms. For them, freedom from Norplant was worth the pain of self-surgery without anesthestics.

There is no need for "sentimental reverie" over lost history in looking at the speculum, as J. Chassar Moir romantically suggests in the epigraph to this chapter. If we do gaze at the "curious speculum," we will catch much more than "a fleeting glimpse of an old hut in Alabama and seven Negro women who suffered, and endured, and had rich reward." We will not only see that slavery served medicine, but we will also see that poor women, particularly poor women of color, continue to serve medicine. Meanwhile medical technologies serve those in power, be they slave owners or concerned taxpayers. By gazing into the "curious speculum," we might consider just how gynecology positions poor women of color and women in general and how it is decided just who is a fitting subject for medical experimentation and display. Gazing into the speculum reminds us to question the politics of visibility, of what is made visible—heroes and obstacles, ringmasters and silver sutures, cervixes and vaginas for surgical manipulation—and what is left invisible—pain and suffering, power differences, slave identities, questionable origins, semi-visible contraceptive technologies. By gazing into the speculum, we may consider how this tool may have solidified the medical institution's involvement in racist, eugenicist practices concerned with the reproductive capacities of poor women.

Gaze into the "curious" speculum. Look again and again and again and reflect on the formation of the medical specialty called gynecology.

3 Cadavers, Dolls, and Prostitutes:
Medical Pedagogy and the Pelvic Rehearsal

My first question, as I suspect yours may be, was, "What *kind* of woman lets four or five novice medical students examine her?" —James G. Blythe, M.D.[1]

Fearing the Unknown

In a paper entitled "The First Pelvic Examination: Helping Students Cope with Their Emotional Responses," printed in the *Journal of Medical Education* in 1979, Julius Buchwald, M.D., a psychiatrist, shares his findings after ten years of conducting seminars with medical students starting their training in OB/GYN.[2] He locates six primary fears associated with a first pelvic examination: (1) "hurting the patient"; (2) "being judged inept"; (3) the "inability to recognize pathology"; (4) "sexual arousal"; (5) "finding the examination unpleasant"; and (6) the "disturbance of the doctor-patient relationship" (when a patient reminded them of somebody they knew, e.g., mother or sister).

Because the pelvic exam produces fear and anxiety in medical students, numerous methods have been used to offer them a pelvic exam "rehearsal." This practice performance is meant to help soothe or disavow student fears while allowing them to practice manual skills. The types of practice performances adopted reveal and promote specific ideas about female bodies and sexuality held by the medical institution. The use of gynecology teaching associates

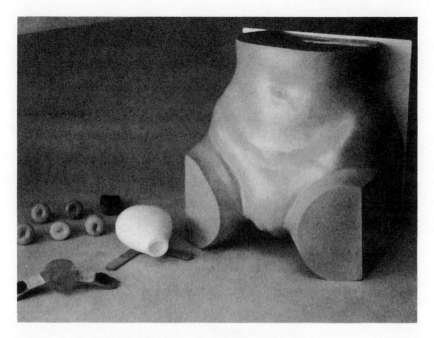

Figure 6. Eva™ Gynecological Manikin. In *Childbirth Graphics* 1, 1996.

(GTAS), trained lay women who teach students using their own bodies, is a relatively new addition to pelvic exam pedagogy that will be examined at length.
Previous to and contemporaneous with this practice, medical schools have cast
a variety of characters as subjects of this pelvic exam rehearsal, including actual
patients, cadavers, anesthetized women, prostitutes, and plastic manikins such
as "Gynny," "Betsi," and "Eva" (see Figure 6). The ways medical students have
been taught to perform pelvic exams illustrate the predicament of the gynecological scenario, a situation in which a practitioner must, by definition, examine
a woman's genitals in a clinical and necessarily nonsexual manner. The array of
pedagogical methods used to teach pelvic exams reveals how the medical institution views female bodies, female sexuality, and the treatment of women.

In pelvic exams, physicians-to-be are confronted with both female genital
display and manipulation, two highly charged cultural acts. If students have previously engaged in gazing at or touching female genitals, most likely they have
done so as a private sexual act (e.g., male students engaging in heterosexual activities and female students masturbating or engaging in lesbian activities). Occasionally there are male or female students who, for a variety of reasons, have
had little or no exposure to naked female bodies, and their fears often revolve

around a fear of the "unknown," which in the case of women's genitals takes the form of a particularly stigmatized mystery.

Students seem to find it very difficult to consider female genital display and manipulation in the medical context as entirely separate from sexual acts and their accompanying fears. Buchwald's list of fears makes explicit the perceived connection between a pelvic examination and a sexual act. "A fear of the inability to recognize pathology" also reflects a fear of contracting a sexually transmitted disease, an actual worry expressed by some of Buchwald's student doctors. Likewise, "a fear of sexual arousal" makes explicit the connection between the pelvic exam and various sexual acts. Buchwald notes that both men and women are subject to this fear of sexual arousal. "A fear of being judged inept" signals a kind of "performance anxiety," a feeling common in both inexperienced and experienced clinical and sexual performers. "A fear of the disturbance of the doctor-patient relationship" recognizes the existence of a type of "incest taboo" within the pelvic exam scenario. Buchwald shares anecdotes of students feeling sick or uncomfortable if the patient being examined reminded them of their mother or sister. Buchwald's work deviates from most publications dealing with the topic of medical students and pelvic exams. Largely, any acknowledgment of this precarious relationship between pelvic exams and sex acts is relatively private and informal, taking place in conversations between students, residents, and doctors, sometimes leaking into private patient interactions. For example, as a student in the 1960s, a male physician was told by the male OB/GYN resident in charge, "During your first 70 pelvic exams, the only anatomy you'll feel is your own." Cultural attitudes about women and their bodies are not checked at the hospital door. If women are largely marketed as sexualized objects of the gaze, why should a gynecological scenario necessarily produce different meanings?

Rehearsing Pelvics

Teaching medical practices is the act of constructing medical realities. In other words, the student is continuously learning by lecture and example what is right and acceptable and, conversely, what is wrong and unacceptable in medical practice. The intractability of medical teaching from medical practice is built into the very title of Foucault's *Birth of the Clinic*. The translator's note recognizes the importance of the choice of the word "clinic": "When Foucault speaks of *la clinique*, he is thinking of both clinical medicine and of the teaching hospital so if one wishes to retain the unity of the concept, one is obliged to use the rather odd-sounding clinic."[3] Medical pedagogy, including textbooks (the focus of the following chapter) and experiential learning, is symbiotic with medical practice; the two work together in the formation, transferal, and perpetuation of medical knowledge. With regard to pelvic exams, this medical knowledge has been acquired in a number of ways.

Many medical students have encountered their first performance of a pelvic exam on an actual patient. Oftentimes a group of students on rounds would repeat pelvic exams one after another on a chosen patient while the attending physician watched. If we consider that the pelvic exam is often sexualized by novice practitioners, this pedagogical situation resembles a "gang rape." Many times there is little communication with the woman being examined, nor is her explicit consent necessarily requested. Due to the intimidation of the medical institution, a woman may not resist repeated examination, even if she is adamantly against the use of her body for pedagogical purposes. This actual patient situation is one that Buchwald locates as anxiety provoking for the medical student (he fails to mention the anxiety this may cause the woman being examined).[4] This situation adds to what Buchwald refers to as the student's "fear of being judged inept": "a frequent remark was, 'if the resident sees the way I'm going about it, he'll think I'm stupid.' In some respects what began to evolve was the image of the experienced, wise, worldly, and sexually competent adult (the resident or attending physician) sneering at the floundering explorations of an adolescent (the medical student) who is striving to become a 'man.' "[5] Buchwald's reading of this situation is gendered inasmuch as he compares the pelvic exam to an adolescent male rite of passage. This gendered reading is telling. The medical apparatus, particularly this 1970s version, incorporates specifically gendered male positions of physician and medical student. Even though there are increasing numbers of women medical students, physicians, and medical educators, the structures of this apparatus, specifically the structures of medical pedagogy, are in many instances unchanged or slow in changing and require a female medical student to fit into this masculinized subject position. Her relationship to this ascribed subject position, particularly as a medical student, may be uncomfortable, as she may be split between identifying with the woman pelvic patient (as she herself has most likely undergone such exams) and with her newly forming role as masculinized spectator. As a medical educator, I frequently witness such a split in female medical students. As Laura Mulvey describes, "trans-sex identification is a *habit* that very easily becomes *second nature*. However, this Nature does not sit easily and shifts restlessly in its borrowed transvestite clothes."[6] Although Mulvey is discussing female cinematic spectatorship, her words are applicable to female medical spectatorship as well. While the anxieties located and described by Buchwald as very "male" in nature may be the very same anxieties experienced by a female medical student, these anxieties take on different twists and meanings with female physicians-in-training.

Other than the attending physician, one person within the pelvic equation who might also judge the student as inept or whose presence might distract the student from performing a proper first exam and therefore cause the student anxiety, is the patient herself. Cadavers, anesthetized women, and anthropomorphic pelvic models like the plastic manikins "Gynny," "Betsi," and "Eva" are pelvic exam subjects who, for a variety of reasons, are rendered absent and therefore cannot talk back or have an opinion about the medical student's performance. These female models alleviate anxiety regarding inappropriate patient performance since they cannot possibly act out. The pedagogical use of these models may also have been developed in order to avert other student fears. If the woman's body is anesthetized, dead, or replaced altogether by a plastic model certainly there can be no fear of causing her pain. However, this logic is questionable in the case of the anesthetized patient: How might repeated pelvic exams under anesthestic affect how a woman "feels" both psychologically and physically when she wakens?

More importantly, the legality of this practice is extremely questionable. How many women would actually consent to this practice? Many women are anxious at the thought of a single pelvic exam, let alone multiple exams. Furthermore, the fear of a pelvic exam is often associated with feeling vulnerable and out of control; under anesthestic, a woman is particularly vulnerable and out of control. And yet teaching medical students how to do pelvic exams on anesthetized women appears to be widely practiced, although public discussion of this method outside (and inside) the medical community is relatively scarce.[7] At a 1979 conference sponsored by the Women's Medical Associations of New York City and State, New Jersey, and Connecticut held at Cornell University Medical College, this issue was discussed and found its way into the *New York Times*, where the conference recommendation was quoted: "If examined in the operating room, patients must be told prior to anesthesia that they will be examined by the members of the operating team, including the medical student."[8] Decades later this recommendation is often unheeded. For example, a surgical nurse I interviewed provided a common scenario: "While doing an exam on a woman who is sedated for a urological procedure, a physician may discover that she has a prolapsed uterus. The student or students observing the procedure will then be invited to perform a bi-manual exam on the woman [inserting two fingers in her vagina while pressing on her abdomen] in order to feel her uterus." I have overheard physicians at a prestigious Chicago medical school encouraging students to "get in surgery as much as possible to get pelvic exam practice." The assumption is that students will not be intimidated by an unconscious woman and that the patient will, in addition, have relaxed abdominal muscles, thus permitting easy palpation of her ovaries and uterus. Many physicians have not heard about such "practicing" and are outraged at the suggestion, maintaining that this is medically sanctioned sexual assault. Some physicians who are aware of the practice dodge the questionable issues, maintaining that for some students it is the only way they will learn.

But what *are* students learning in this scenario? By using anesthetized women, cadavers, or plastic models as pelvic exam subjects students are being taught that a model patient (or patient model) is one who is essentially unconscious or backstage to the performance of the pelvic exam; she should be numb to the exam, providing no feedback and offering no opinions. In the tradition of Sims's experiments, passive and powerless female patients are considered ideal "participants" in the learning process. In addition, students practicing on essentially silent and lifeless models are learning that the manual skills associated with completing a pelvic exam are more important than the fundamental skills needed to interact with the patient—skills that ideally would help the patient relax and participate in the exam.

Perhaps these rehearsal methods are used under the assumption that an anesthetized, dead, or plastic model is unerotic and will thus relieve students of Buchwald's fear #4, "a fear of sexual arousal." And yet the rendering of the object of manipulation or the gaze as passive simply heightens the power differential between examiner and examined that can in effect tap into an altogether different system of erotics. Necrophilia may be coded into a pelvic examination on a cadaver. Similarly, there have been noted cases of sexual abuse when patients are under anesthetic.[9] Likewise, the anthropomorphically named pelvic manikins "Gynny," "Betsi," and "Eva," with their custom orifices for medical penetration, could be recognized as the medical correlates to inflatable sex dolls.[10]

In the late 1970s, numerous medical pedagogues were reexamining what one physician referred to as "the time-honored methods" of pelvic exam pedagogy: students examining anesthetized women, conscious patients, cadavers, or plastic models.[11] The problems with these methods were discussed in a number of articles. The authors of the 1977 article "Professional Patients: An Improved Method of Teaching Breast and Pelvic Examination" in the *Journal of Reproductive Medicine* found that training medical students on actual patients "has many disadvantages, including infringement of patients' rights, inadequate feedback and moral and ethical concerns. Another approach that is widely used is the anesthetized preoperative patient. Again, problems include informed consent, increased cost and/or risk and lack of an interpersonal exchange. The introduction of the 'Gynny' and 'Betsi' models has been an attempt at improvement, but not without drawbacks, which include a lack of personal communication, unreal exposure and difficulty with 'live' correlation."[12] Where was the medical community to find these living models? Some went to what must have seemed a very natural source. In the early 1970s a number of schools, including the University of Washington Medical School and the University of Oklahoma Physician's Associate Program, hired prostitutes to serve as "patient simulators."[13] What other women would accept payment for spreading their legs? Logically, these educators felt that a prostitute would be the most fitting *kind* of woman for the job. In a sense, the patriarchal medical establishment took the position of a rich uncle, paying for his nephew, the medical student, to have his first sexual experience with a prostitute. This gendered suggestion assumes that female medical students are structurally positioned as masculinized "nephew" subjects as well.

Although lip service has been paid to the supposed importance of desexualizing the pelvic patient, in choosing prostitute patient models, medical educators inadvertently situated the exam as a sexualized act. They must have thought that only a prostitute would voluntarily submit to exams repeatedly and for nondiagnostic purposes. Or perhaps the underlying assumption was that a lady *pays* to get examined whereas a whore *gets paid* for the same exam. It may have also been assumed that prostitutes are more accustomed to and have a higher tolerance for vaginal pain than other women and would thus be more fitting practice models for novice students. In choosing to hire prostitutes as patients the boundaries of pornographic and medical practice were collapsed. Within this scenario of a hired prostitute, the student physician was put in the position of a medicalized lover or "john." Certainly Buchwald's fear #3, "a fear of sexual arousal," was confirmed and even encouraged by hiring prostitutes. Buchwald notes that certain students "appeared to project their anxiety by asking, 'what should I do if the patient starts responding sexually?' "[14] By hiring prostitutes as pelvic patients, the medical establishment not only enforced the trope of the "seductive patient," but also paid for it.[15] "Playing doctor" in this pelvic rehearsal cast with patient prostitutes threatened to translate the pelvic exam into an act of sexualized penetration and bodily consumption.

In many cases when prostitutes were hired, the medical student was led to believe that the woman being examined was a clinical outpatient rather than a prostitute. Thus the prostitute still had a relatively passive position in the training of medical students. In order to properly perform her role as clinical outpatient, she could offer the student little feedback. In addition, the working logic of the medical educators remained relatively opaque inasmuch as the student was not directly learning about the medical establishment's opinion of model patients. And yet these attitudes undoubtedly found their way into medical practice. Years later, students are still told by certain unaware medical faculty that GTAS are prostitutes. Today certain faculty still conclude that no other *kind* of woman would submit her body to multiple exams in exchange for a fee. This points to the importance of understanding the recent history of pelvic pedagogy. Those physicians trained in the 1970s are the same physicians practicing and educating today.

Some physicians found fault with the use of prostitutes as pelvic models. According to the authors of "Utilization of Simulated Patients to Teach the Routine Pelvic Examination," "the employment of prostitute patient simulators is not satisfactory. The prostitutes employed by the PA (Physician's Associate) program were not articulate enough to provide the quality of instructive feedback necessary for an optimal educational experience. Their employment was costly at $25 per hour, and that expense prohibited their extensive and long-term use. Also, and more importantly prostitutes had abnormal findings on examination prior to their utilization."[16] Pathology was not desirable in these model patients: in the pelvic rehearsal, students were not to be distracted by abnormal findings. Rather, the patient simulator needed to be standardized as normal like the plastic model. In addition, the prostitute was expensive. She received market value for her bodily consumption, unlike the income-free corpse, indebted actual patient, and the cut-rate graduate students that the authors of the article hired at $10 per hour. And although prostitutes did offer some student critique (comments such as "poor introduction," "too serious," "too rough," and "forgot to warm the speculum") their language skills were not medically acceptable.[17] What the medical establishment needed was a model who could engage in medicalese, was more cost efficient, and had normal, healthy anatomy. The GTA would be the answer.

The GTA Program

In 1968 at the University of Iowa Medical School's Department of Obstetrics and Gynecology, Dr. Robert Kretzschmar instituted a new method for teaching junior medical students how to perform the pelvic exam.[18] For the pelvic model he used a "simulated patient," first defined in the medical literature as a "person who has been trained to completely simulate a patient or any aspect of a patient's illness depending upon the educational need."[19] Many simulated patients were actresses and actors hired by the medical establishment to realistically portray a patient. Their critical feedback was not traditionally requested. They simply served as a warm body for the practicing student. This stage of Kretzschmar's program was not dissimilar to the other programs that hired prostitutes. Initially, Kretzschmar adhered to this simulated patient model. He hired a nurse for the role of patient. She agreed to repeated exams by medical students; "however, it was necessary to compromise open communication with her, as she was draped at her request in such a way as to remain anonymous."[20] The curtain rose but the nurse's knowledge, thoughts, feelings, and face remained backstage. All that was revealed was the object of the exam: the woman's pelvic region. The logic behind draping the simulated patient presumed that if "only a whore gets paid" for a nondiagnostic exam, perhaps the nurse could avoid whore status by becoming faceless and silent.

In many gynecology textbooks, as will be examined in the following chapter, a similar logic prevails. Photographs picturing women are cropped so that faces are not shown or bands are placed across eyes to maintain the model's anonymity. If the woman's face and eyes are pictured, the photo could enter the realm of pornography; the woman imaged cannot be soliciting or meeting the medical practitioner's gaze, a potentially sexualized act. If the nurse who served as simulated patient was draped to maintain her anonymity she was in effect attempting to desexualize her body for the medical gaze. But is this an effective strategy for the desexualization of the exam? Is a faceless, vulnerable female body less erotic? In addition, although this professional patient model rehearsal did save actual patients from the task of performing the role of pelvic model, it did little to encourage communication between student and patient. Maintaining such anonymity taught the students that it was acceptable and even preferable for them to ignore the woman backstage behind the drape. They were also shown that a modest woman, unlike a prostitute, would need to disassociate her face from her body. And therefore, a modest woman preferred to be treated as though she were anonymous and invisible.

In 1972, Kretzschmar instituted a different program. The new simulated patient, now named the gynecology teaching associate (GTA), would serve as both patient and instructor, stressing the importance of communication skills in addition to teaching the manual skills required to perform a proper pelvic exam. Unlike the nurse clinician who was first hired as a simulated patient in 1968, the GTA would actively teach and offer feedback to medical students, forsaking any anonymity through draping. The GTAs first hired by Kretzschmar were women who were working on or had received advanced degrees in the behavioral sciences but who had no formal medical training. The women had normal, healthy anatomy and were willing to undergo multiple exams. They then received elaborate instruction in female anatomy and physiology, pelvic and breast examination, self-breast-examination and abdominal examination, with an emphasis on normal anatomy. They worked in pairs, one GTA serving as "patient" TA, one as "instructor" TA. They were assigned a small group of medical students and conducted the educational session in an exam room. The "patient" TA received the exam, role-playing as patient and co-instructor, while the "instructor" TA remained alongside the students, helping and instructing them during the exam. After receiving two exams the "patient" TA changed from gown to street clothes and became "instructor" TA, and the "instructor" TA changed from street clothes to gown to become the "patient" TA. The teaching session was then repeated with a new group of medical students, thus assuring that one TA of each pair would not receive all the exams.

Kretzschmar's GTA model provided a radically new way of teaching medical students how to do pelvic and breast exams. No longer was the simulated patient a teaching tool; now she was both teacher and patient. The women's movement undoubtedly influenced this model. In the 1960s and '70s women were demanding better health care and some took matters into their own hands by establishing self-help groups and feminist clinics. In fact, many early GTAS were directly associated with these groups and clinics and believed their new position within the medical establishment as GTA could allow them to bring their alternative knowledge to the heart of the beast.

Kretzschmar received a variety of critical responses from the medical community for his new GTA program. Some were positive, applauding him for his innovative method and his success in avoiding a "men's club" attitude by hiring women as teachers.[21] Some, however, were skeptical at best. They were particularly cautious regarding the GTAS' motives for participating in such a perverse endeavor. The epigraph to this chapter—"What *kind* of woman lets four or five novice medical students examine her?"—was a question asked by many physicians, according to Kretzschmar. Some human subjects committee members who reviewed the GTA concept "felt that women who were willing to participate must be motivated by one or more of several questionable needs, such as desperate financial circumstances (in which case exploiting their need would be unethical). Others fear the women would be exhibitionists or that they would use the pelvic exam to serve some perverse internal sexual gratification (in which case portraying them as normal to medical students would be irresponsible)."[22] Once again, the pelvic exam was compared to a sexual act by the medical establishment. Cultural fears regarding female sexuality and its perversions surface in these objections to the GTA program. Only a nymphomaniac would seek out multiple exams, enjoying repeated penetration with speculums and fingers. Also, poor women might lower themselves to such embodied work out of desperation, thereby aligning the GTA with the prostitute in an explanatory narrative. Furthermore, the committee questioned the psychological stability of the GTA, with the assumption "that women who are emotionally unstable might be attracted to the program, or that undergoing repeated examination might be psychologically harmful."[23] These human subject committee members reveal their nineteenth-century ideas about (white) women: frail female psychological health and sexual health are seen as mutually dependent and delicate partners. If their equilibrium is tipped by the "pleasure" or pain incurred by the excessive sexualized act of multiple pelvic exams, then who knows what horrors will take place.

Unquestionably, teaching female genital display and manipulation has been the cause of a great deal of anxiety. These fears are much more reflective of the medical institution's constructions of the female psyche and female sexuality than of any actual threat to women posed by the role of GTA. One reason the role of GTA could seem threatening to these critics is that they were faced with a new and potentially powerful position for women in the predominantly male medical establishment. Their attempt at pathologizing the GTA could have been propelled by a desire to maintain the status quo: that *normal* women are passive, quiet, disembodied recipients of a hopelessly unpleasant but necessary pelvic exam. For them, perhaps this was the least threatening alternative.

Despite its early critics, Kretzschmar's model has become the pedagogical norm in the vast majority of institutions. Over 90 percent of North American medical schools employ this instructional method, recognized as "excellent" by the Association of Professors of Gynecology and Obstetrics Undergraduate Education Committee.[24] Many GTA programs throughout the country maintain the same basic form as Kretzschmar's 1972 incarnation, though there is some variation. For example, some schools have GTAs working alone, rather than in pairs; a few schools still hire the more passive live pelvic model or "professional patient" to be used in conjunction with an instructing physician. The use of pelvic manikins, anesthetized women, cadavers, and actual patients continues to supplement some student learning.

Beginning in 1988, I was employed as a GTA by the University of Illinois at Chicago (UIC) medical school. Periodically, I also taught at two other Chicago-area medical schools and in one physician's assistant program. Excepting one institution, all my teaching experiences have followed Kretzschmar's GTA model. For the institution that had not adopted Kretzschmar's model, I worked as a "professional patient." A physician or nurse-midwife served as instructor, and I was hired primarily to model the exam for three students and the instructor. Whenever a clinician-instructor was unable to attend, I volunteered to work as both instructor and model, adopting a variation of Kretzschmar's model.

In discussing the GTA, I will collapse the roles of instructor and patient GTA into a single role. While this is reductive of the complexity of the partner relationship assumed by the instructor and patient GTAS, it may help clarify their common mission. And indeed many schools have collapsed the roles of the two GTAS into a single GTA who is paired with three or four students. After years of teaching, I find this to be a better model. It is impossible for students to position the instructor as silent patient if she is the only educator in the room. When there is a single teacher who also serves as "patient" students are faced with the jarring experience of examining a woman who knows more about gynecological exam than they do.

The Teaching Session

The students enter the exam room, where the GTA wears a patient gown. She is both their teacher and the object of their examination. The GTA explains the purpose of the teaching session. She is a healthy woman with normal anatomy who is there to help the students learn how to perform a proper breast and pelvic exam. Medical students, however, have been indoctrinated into a system that privileges pathology. They have learned that what is normal and healthy is not as interesting as what is abnormal and unhealthy. Some students seem disappointed when they are told that the GTA session is one part of their medical education in which they will not be presented with pathology.

The GTA explains that the patient, performed by herself, is there for a yearly exam. She has no complaints. Rather, they are there to have the experience of examining a normal, healthy woman and thus should offer the "patient" feedback after each part of the exam, letting her know that "everything appears healthy and normal." The GTA emphasizes that no woman can hear the phrase "healthy and normal" too much. For many medical students "healthy" and "normal" are new additions to their medical script. Often, these second- and third-year medical students admit that the GTA session is the first time they have been encouraged to use these words. In a moment that struck me as simultaneously encouraging and tragicomic, one student, upon hearing me discuss the phrase "healthy and normal," pulled a 3 x 5 notecard and pen out of his pocket. He then said, "Tell me those words again. I want to write them down so I can remember them." In medical pedagogy, pathology is the norm, and normalcy is often viewed as mundane or unremarkable. For a woman in need of her yearly pap smear, the clinician's preoccupation with pathology can have sad consequences, both adding to the woman's anxiety about the possibility of the clinician finding that something is wrong and leaving her with the feeling that something is wrong regardless of actual clinical findings.

During the GTA session, other aspects of the students' scripts are rewritten and relearned. They are taught to use words that are less sexually connotative or awkward. For example, "I am going to *examine* your breasts now" as opposed to "I'm going to *feel* your breasts now." A number of script adjustments are made: "insert" or "place" the speculum as opposed to "stick in"; "healthy and normal" as opposed to "looks great." Changes are encouraged with regard to tool names: "footrests" as opposed to "stirrups"; "bills" rather than "blades" of the speculum.

When I was working as a "professional patient" with a young white woman physician as instructor, she kept referring to the "blades" of the speculum while teaching the students. I explained to her that many people within the medical community were replacing the term "blades" with "bills" because of the obvious violent connotations of the term, especially given that it refers to that part of the speculum placed inside the woman's body. The physician replied, agitated, "Well, we don't say it to the *patient*." Her assumption was that words that circulate within the medical community do not affect patient care or physician attitudes toward patients as long as those words do not reach the patient's ears. This is naive and faulty thinking, resistant to change, disabling the idea that language does indeed help structure attitudes and practice.

Furthermore, in that scenario I *was* the patient and the word "blade" was being used to refer to the part of an instrument that was to be placed inside *my* body. My thoughts were largely ignored even though I was hired to perform the role of patient. For the rest of the session, the physician begrudgingly used the word "bills," looking at me and punching the word each time she used it. Weeks later I worked at the same institution with a young white male physician whose language was considerate and carefully chosen and who continually encouraged my feedback and participation within the session. He consistently referred to the "bills" of the speculum of his own accord. By seeking out a patient's opinion and input within both a teaching situation and an actual exam, the clinician is relinquishing a portion of control and offering the patient more power within the exam scenario. As is evident in these two examples, gender does not necessarily determine a clinician's attitudes toward patients or the patient model.

The GTA offers many tips on how the clinician may help the patient feel more powerful and less frightened during an exam. "Talk before touch" is a technique used in the pelvic exam by which the clinician lets the patient know that she or he is about to examine the patient: with the phrase "You'll feel my hand now," the clinician applies the the back of her or his hand to the more neutral space of the insides of a patient's thighs. Since the patient cannot *see* where the clinician's hands are, this technique offers her important information about where and when she will be touched.

Eye contact is another important and often ignored part of the pelvic exam. The GTA reminds the student to maintain eye contact with her throughout most parts of the exam. Many women complain that oftentimes clinicians have spoken at their genitals or breasts rather than to them. Eye contact not only offers the clinician another diagnostic tool, since discomfort and pain are often expressed in a patient's face, but it also makes the patient feel as though she is being treated as a person rather than as fragmented parts. In order to facilitate eye contact, the students are taught to raise the table to a 45-degree angle rather than leaving it flat. This has the added benefit of relaxing the woman's abdominal muscles. Specific draping techniques are taught so that the student-clinician cannot hide in front of the drape, ignoring the parts of the woman that reside backstage behind the curtain.

Given that the medical institution routinely segments and dissects bodies for examination, maintaining eye contact with the patient is often difficult for students. Considering the sexual overtones of this particular exam, many students (and practitioners) find it very difficult to meet their patient's gaze. Likewise, there are patients who will not look into their examiner's eyes due to shame or embarrassment or a desire to be "invisible." While this is always a possibility, the GTA asserts that the practitioner must initiate eye contact even if the patient declines the offer, so that the patient at least has a choice of whether to "look back" at the clinician.

Similarly, the GTA encourages students to continuously communicate with the patient, informing her as to what they are doing, how they are doing it, and why they are doing it. For example, the student must show the woman the speculum, holding it high enough so that she can see it (without aiming it at her like a gun), while explaining, "This is a speculum. I will insert this part, the bills, into your vagina, opening them so that I can see your cervix, the neck of your uterus. I do this so that I can take a pap smear, which is a screening test for cervical cancer." Many women have had dozens of pelvic exams without ever having had the opportunity to see a speculum. More often, they hear the clanking of metal as the speculum is snuck out of its drawer and into their vagina.

Clinicians should not use words that patients will not understand, nor should they patronize patients; rather, they should piggyback medical terms with simpler phrases. In addition, students are taught that women should be given verbal instruction when they need to move or undress. For example, the woman should not be handled like a limp doll as a clinician removes her gown for the breast exam; instead the woman should be asked to remove her own gown. This helps her feel a little more in control of her own body and space. Ideally, the pelvic exam can become an educational session and the patient a partner in her own exam.

Lilla Wallis, M.D., an OB/GYN professor at Cornell University Medical School and a strong advocate of the GTA program, promotes this idea of "the patient as partner in the pelvic exam,"[25] and in addition encourages the use of many techniques popular within the women's health movement. Wallis adopts what some institutions might consider radical techniques. For instance, she urges clinicians to offer patients a hand mirror so that they might see what is being done to them. The patient is encouraged to look at her own genitals and not feel as though this were a view limited to the practitioner. Wallis also questions the draping of the patient: "This separates the patient from her own body. It suggests that the genitals are a forbidden part of her body that she should modestly ignore. It also isolates the doctor."[26] Instead, she believes that patients should have the choice of whether to be draped or not. She refers to the use of GTAS as "a quiet revolution" in American medical schools, believing that GTA programs will lead to better, more thoughtful care by physicians.

Is the rehearsal with GTAS enough to change medical attitudes about women, female sexuality, and women's bodies? Can the use of GTAS actually affect these attitudes? While I was working as a "professional patient" or "model" at an esteemed Chicago-area medical school, an interesting sequence of events happened that pointed out to me the vast difference between teaching students as a GTA and serving as a "model." The physician I was to be working with was delayed at a meeting, so I started working with the four medical students. I stressed patient communication, helping the woman relax, "talk before touch," and educating the woman during the exam. The students were responsive, as the vast majority of students are, understanding my explanations for why these techniques were important and making an effort to adopt them as they made their way through the breast and pelvic exam.

I had finished teaching all four students how to do a breast exam and two students had completed pelvic exams, when the physician, a young white man, rushed in, apologizing for being late. He then proceeded to contradict much of what I had taught the students. I argued my points, but he insisted that many women were not interested in explanations or education but just "wanted it to be over with." He taught students a one-handed technique so that only one hand ever got "dirty," leaving the other hand free. He basically ignored my presence, so much so that at one point I had to dislodge his elbow, which was digging into my thigh as he leaned over, bracing himself on me, to see if my cervix was in view. The two remaining students were visibly more nervous than the students who had already had their turns. They were rushed and forgot "talk before touch" in an attempt to incorporate the shortcuts that the physician had taught them.

At the end of the session, he encouraged the students to get into surgery to examine as much pathology as possible: "I have an 18cm uterus I'll be working on. Come by." I pictured this enlarged uterus alone on a surgical table without its woman-encasement. He assured the students, "The only way you're going to learn what is normal is to see a lot of pathology." I had emphasized the wide variety of what is normal, how vulvas were all different and that students would need to see a lot of normal anatomy to understand what was not normal. After this physician's intrusion, the lone female medical student in the group kept looking at me at each point the physician contradicted me. She smiled at me empathetically, understanding the severity of the emotional and political sabotage I must have been feeling as both an educator and a naked woman "patient." Before the students left, three of the four shook my hand, genuinely thanking me for helping them. The one student who had been resistant to some of the techniques I had taught them was more suspicious. He said to me sternly, "Can I ask you, what are your motivations for doing this?"

The View from the Table

Implicit in the role of the GTA is a fundamental contradiction. On the one hand, she is an educator, more knowledgeable than medical students about pelvic and breast exams although she holds no medical degree. In this sense she is in a position of power, disseminating various truths about the female body and its examination. On the other hand, the GTA is bound to a traditionally vulnerable and powerless lithotomy position: lying on her back, heels in footrests. Oftentimes, her body is viewed as the true learning tool, with her words taking a back seat to this "hands-on" educational experience. In an interview, one GTA expressed her frustration: "Sometimes I feel like it's strange being nice, being like an airline hostess of the body. For example [she points two fingers as stewardesses do at cabin exits], 'Now we're coming to the *mons pubis*.' You have to be nice. I've seen some GTAS who were strong and businesslike about it, and I don't feel comfortable doing that but it's a strain having to be nice." This is a beautiful metaphor for describing the GTA's predicament: She is there to make medical students comfortable as they journey across the female body. Comparing the GTA to an airline hostess highlights the pink-collar service role she performs: she is working for the medical school in a position that only women can fill and she is there to make the students feel less apprehensive and more knowledgeable. The fact that she needs to be "nice" while presenting her own body points to one of the performative aspects of the GTA's role as educator. Like the stewardess, the GTA is costumed with a smile, a well-defined script, and a uniform.

In her book *The Managed Heart: Commercialization of Human Feeling*, Arlie

Russell Hochschild connects Marx's factory worker to the flight attendant; both must "mentally detach themselves—the factory worker from his own body and physical labor, and the flight attendant from her own feelings and emotional labor."[27] The case of the GTA becomes an interesting blend of these two types of alienation. She is like the flight attendant in that she manages her own feelings, what the GTA above calls "being nice." She must learn how to deal with the occasional hostile or overtly sexual medical student customer. She is there to make the student's trip through the female body comfortable, safe, and enjoyable. But it is her own body, not the meal tray or the fuselage of the airplane, that she is presenting to the paying customer.[28] In this sense, the GTA is like Marx's factory laborer who uses his own body. She is getting paid for her body's use-value in the production of a trained medical student.

Structurally, with regard to physical labor and the management of feelings, the GTA resides in a position similar to that of a prostitute. Both GTAs and prostitutes sell the use of their body for what may be loosely termed "educational purposes." Both must manage their feelings, acting the part of willing recipient to probing instruments. Medical school history aside, GTAs and prostitutes have a good deal in common. This is perhaps why numerous GTAs have remarked on their husband's or partner's discomfort with their work. Certainly not all GTAs have partners who consider their teaching to be a sexual act and so object to or are threatened by it. But partner discontent is not uncommon. One GTA explains, "My boyfriend had problems with my teaching when I first moved in with him. It didn't bother him before I was living with him. I moved in only a couple of months before we got married and then he started voicing his complaints. . . . I think they [significant others] are afraid it's sexual and I think the students are afraid it's sexual. They're afraid about how they're going to react, whether they're going to be aroused, but it's so clinical." Another GTA present at this interview said she had a similar problem in that her boyfriend was "concerned" and "uneasy": "I said to him if you're going to give me $150 to sit with you or have sex with you or whatever, fine, otherwise I'm going to make my money."

GTAS' partners are not the only ones who have been distressed by the GTA role. Some early women's health activists expressed a different kind of uneasiness as they quickly realized the pink-collar nature of the job. When the GTA program was first starting in the 1970s, these feminist health activists participating in the project sensed that they were still expected to mimic a patriarchal medical performance, employing language, techniques, and attitudes that reinforced the established power differential between pelvic exam clinician and female patient. These groups felt that working for a medical school did not allow them enough autonomy to teach what were, for them, important exam techniques. They believed that change within the medical establishment was virtually impossible and encouraged women not to participate in pelvic teaching within medical schools.[29] Of these GTAs, some simply discontinued their work with medical students. Others continued teaching self-motivated medical students who would voluntarily visit feminist self-help clinics for continuing education. These feminist teachers regarded this new experience as highly valuable. As one activist notes: "The rapport experienced by the program participants and the [feminist teaching] nurses had been astounding . . . The result was an exploration with students of such topics as sexuality, abortion, contraception and ambivalent feelings regarding their roles."[30] After refusing the medical institution's version of a proper pelvic exam rehearsal, these health activists composed their own.

In his article about medical students' six fears of pelvic exams, Buchwald accepted student fears without either questioning why young physicians-to-be would have such fears or searching for the cultural attitudes underlying them. Indeed, he might have been employing a Freudian psychoanalytic model that would entirely justify such fears: faced with the abject, castrated vulva, medical students *would* be terrified by the exam. These feminist teachers who rejected the GTA program, however, confronted and questioned student fears, realizing the importance of helping these future caregivers shed deep anxieties and ambivalences regarding female bodies. For years, medical pedagogues blatantly sidestepped these issues by employing teaching methods that would simply ignore or Band-aid student fears: hiring prostitutes would confirm student ideas regarding promiscuous female sexuality and its relationship to the pelvic exam; the use of plastic manikins would soothe student fears of touching real female genitals; while the use of anesthetized women and cadavers would present an unconscious "model" patient. Only with the use of GTAs have medical schools attempted to incorporate women patients' thoughts, feelings, and ideas into pelvic exam teaching. And yet, as these feminist teachers pointed out decades ago and as my experiences have occasionally confirmed, it may be impossible to educate students properly within the medical institution given unacknowledged cultural attitudes about female bodies and female sexuality.

The pelvic exam is in itself a pedagogical scenario. The woman receiving the exam, despite the political or philosophical orientation of the clinician, is taught attitudes about female bodies. In this respect, the physician is as much a pedagogue as a healer, if the two roles can be separated. In teaching medical students, one is therefore teaching teachers, transferring knowledge, methods, and attitudes to those practitioners who will in turn conduct private tutorials with individual women who seek their care. Thus the methods used to teach medical students how to do pelvic exams significantly structure how these physicians-to-be will educate their future patients. The various ways medical students have been taught to do pelvic exams are intimately related to the medical institution's attitudes toward women and in turn structure how future practitioners perceive and treat their women patients.

The use of GTAS alters the normal pelvic scenario to some degree. Here the "doctor" is being educated by the "patient," a potentially powerful role for the GTA. As an educator, she may critique the student from the patient's perspective (e.g., "Use less pressure," "you're not palpating the ovary there"). One would think that the medical student would not argue with the woman who is experiencing the exam. And yet, because the GTA is not a physician, the student is sometimes skeptical of her expertise, doubting her advice even if it is based on her bodily experience. The very fact that her experience is bodily may serve to deny the importance of her role. Her embodiment of the exam makes her a curious and suspect educator in the eyes of many since she is being *paid* for the use of her body in addition to her teaching skills. Her role continually elicits questions about what *kind* of woman she must be to undergo multiple exams.

In the GTA's educational performance there is no hypothetical signified, no abstract female body; rather the GTA is a fleshy referent with her own shape, anatomical variation, and secretions. At the site of the GTA, medicine, pornography, and prostitution mingle, highlighting medical attitudes regarding female sexuality, vulvar display, and genital manipulation. The teaching session may be a "representation" of a "real" exam, but for the GTA, as well as the medical student, it is simultaneously representation *and* practice.

It is curious, but not surprising, that the medical institution has focused so much attention on the GTA's role. Instead of focusing on what *kind* of woman would allow multiple exams to be performed on her, physicians might be more justified in asking how the medical establishment perceives the proper pelvic model or model patient. Or to turn the question back onto the medical institution itself, one might ask what *kind* of man or woman will *give* multiple exams. Unless there is a continued investigation of the medical structures that construct and reflect attitudes about female bodies and sexuality, the answer to this question might indeed be something to really fear.

4 Apparent Females and Female Appearances:
On the Status of Genitals in Medical Textbook Illustration

When I was in medical school, a fellow student had never seen a naked woman and would start sweating anytime anybody mentioned a pelvic exam. The time was coming that he would have to do his first exam. A bunch of us bought him a copy of *Penthouse* so he would know what he was going to be looking at. —A female gynecologist

I've sold some of my photos to medical textbooks. I think the publishers got my name from a sex magazine. Once they wanted a photograph of an enlarged clitoris, and I happened to have one—she was even spreading her pussy lips. But they wouldn't take the photo because she had red nail polish on. —Annie Sprinkle

I sit in an esteemed university's medical library, paging through gynecological textbooks, wondering if I will be "caught looking." Without a medical degree or medical school enrollment, I am little more than an illegitimate voyeur. Worst of all, I am hardly even reading the words, I am only gazing at the pictures. Working on this chapter, I am considering how medical images make women's bodies. Specifically, I am interested in the ways medical textbook images negotiate the public presentation of female genitalia. As discussed in the previous chapter, I have worked as a gynecology teaching associate at this very same medical school, teaching medical students how to perform pelvic and breast exams using my body as teaching tool. However, that embodied practice affords me little in the way of legitimate affiliation with the medical institution. Thus I approach these images as an academic outsider, an interloper, but I also come to these textbooks with my experiences as a woman patient and as a GTA; I have been an educator performing the role of patient, subject to the effects of the books' discourses, to their direct production and dissemination of knowledge about the female body. I consider how these textbooks affect the way medical practitioners and students see *my* body. Looking at these books, the division between medical representation and practice seems to melt away. At some level, these texts appear to contain the key to my experiences as a pelvic teacher. Did these books help produce the third-year medical student who needed to write down the words "healthy and normal" on a 3 × 5 card so he could remember them? Were these texts written by the attending physician who contradicted my emphasis on slow, communicative exams, instead urging the students to work fast by not getting both hands "dirty" and to get into surgery to "see as much pathology as possible"? Or maybe it was not *that* attending, but rather *his* attending when *he* was a student who authored one of them? I create fantastic genealogies in my head, linking the various students and staff I have encountered to specific captions and images. I enjoy this game.

It is not simply the naked content of these pictures that produces in me this feeling of illicit or pornographic viewing. In looking at these images, I have the pleasure of trespassing the defined boundaries of the medical sphere, venturing away from my prescribed role as patient or institutional teaching tool, reading medical images without the proper credentials. I enjoy discovering the sources and products of various attitudes toward women's bodies that I have encountered while performing the role of patient body within hospital and clinic walls. I find disquieted pleasure in this critical practice as I leaf through the pages of these large books, gazing at images that are often both very disturbing and critically rich. Here in the library, I feel that my secretive, medically inappropriate mixture of pleasure and displeasure must somehow emanate from my cubicle. Is it just a paranoid fantasy that I continuously expect a passerby to tap me on the shoulder and ask me to leave?

Female privates enter the public as spectacle predominantly in the forms of art, pornography, and medicine. While there is often only a tenuous distinction between the categories of art and pornography, classically, artistic representation has euphemized or metaphorized female genitalia, picturing them as a smooth lack, devoid of pubic hair or any other indication of something to be seen.[1] Pornographic representations, like gynecological representations, often clearly depict female genitals, making a spectacle out of the usually hidden vulva. In gynecological textbooks, female genitalia *must* be pictured; the very discipline of gynecology depends upon exposing the vulva. Since gynecology and pornography often represent exposed vulvas, there is always the possibility that a representation in one sphere may exceed its boundaries and find itself within another domain. For example, one could masturbate while looking at an erotic medical image or study an unobscured pornographic representation for physiological information, thus drawing them back and forth across the imaginary border between science and pornography. These slippages are evident in the epigraphs to this chapter; medical students purchased mainstream pornography in order to view female genitals in preparation for a gynecology rotation and medical publishers sought out a porn star–photographer in order to solicit specific medical images. From an institutional standpoint, there can be costs to such transgressions. For pornographers, the clinical pornographic image may lose its eroticism. For medical publishers, as in the case of those who rejected Annie Sprinkle's images because of the model's red-polished nails, the erotic medical image may endanger the "objectivity" of the sacrosanct medical sphere.[2] But this danger does not preclude the use of pornography for the education of medical students or the porn industry's use of medical tropes for titillation.[3]

Pornography, as both a representational practice and a category, challenges the institutional sanctity of medicine, constantly taunting and exposing its vulnerability, particularly in the realm of gynecological images. However, the display of pathology fills a very particular role with regard to gynecological images. Pathology serves to mediate the pornographic possibilities in medical imagery, reminding the viewer that the pleasures of viewing the patient body pictured are not about imaging the potential sex object, but rather about imaging the potential medical object.[4] Because of the visibility of pathology, the body is coded as suitable for medical visualization, penetration, and therefore clinical intervention. The sighting of pathology defines the desirable medical object. Likewise, the pictorial presentation of pathology simultaneously serves as the visible evidence of potential clinical success and limits the possibility of pornographic readings of images.

These ideas will be made clearer through a close reading of images found in a preeminent obstetrics and gynecology textbook. Edited by four male ob-gyns, *Danforth's Obstetrics and Gynecology* is a commonly used medical textbook. Says editor James R. Scott, M.D.: "Since the publication of the first edition in 1966, *Danforth's Obstetrics and Gynecology* has been widely acclaimed as a standard textbook for medical students, house officers, and practicing physicians. For many of us it has formed the basis of learning and reference in our specialty."

Danforth's is explicitly constructed to belong to the medical canon: "It is designed to cover the modern practice of obstetrics and gynecology as concisely and completely as possible and with *maximum authority*" (italics mine).[5] *Danforth's* five previous successful editions have even "been translated into several languages and used worldwide." Given its production, distribution, and reception, *Danforth's* is clearly a powerful instrument in the dissemination of knowledge about obstetrics, gynecology, and the female body.

Undoubtedly, the images in *Danforth's* play a significant role in the editors' presentation of scientific truths about the female body. This visual presentation of the specificities of female bodies is part of a larger, more general tradition of seeking knowledge about the human body, particularly about human sexual difference and sexuality. In her book *Hard Core*, Linda Williams links cinematic hard core to this very tradition, which she labels *scientia sexualis*, borrowing the title from Foucault. Williams discusses Charcot's photographic record of female hysteria in order to note "the extent the scientific will-to-knowledge of the female body is already intersected by the solicitation of a pleasurable and prurient show." She then asserts, "But we should not forget that the reverse is also true: the emerging visual pleasures of the late-nineteenth-century frenzy of the visible remain wedded to the scientific will-to-knowledge."[6] Given this historical framework, it is possible to conceive of both gynecological images and pornography as truth-seeking texts, aimed at isolating the "truth of sex." Thus Williams helps provide an explanation for the epigraphs that began this chapter: the medical students purchased *Penthouse* for their peer's own personal "will-to-knowledge," and photographer Annie Sprinkle's pornographic photos were, if properly framed, the kind of truthful documentation sought after by medical textbook editors. Porn texts, like gynecological textbooks, can therefore be seen as part of a larger attempt to know more about human sex and sexuality.

While I would agree with Williams that scientific display of the female body is inevitably "intersected by the solicitation of a pleasurable and prurient show," I wish to consider how contemporary gynecological texts, in particular, attempt to mediate and disavow this inevitability. For instance, in the case of Sprinkle's photograph, the woman's red nail polish transgressed some undefined (but strongly felt) boundary of scientific coding for the editors. Through an examination of images in *Danforth's*, I will consider what constitute the boundaries between pornographic and medical representation. Important to an understanding of these boundaries is a consideration of the types of representation employed in medical textbooks. Concentrating almost entirely on cinematic and photographic representation, Williams links the truth seeking of hard-core images to the mechanistic recording function of the camera. In contemporary gynecological textbooks, photography is enlisted for very specific purposes. Considering the use of photography and other means of representation, namely drawing, in contemporary medical textbooks reveals how the solicitation of a pleasurable and prurient show is mediated for the sake of medicine.

Competing Forms

In *Danforth's*, as in other medical textbooks, images are vital to the construction of medical knowledge. Not simply pictorial illustrations, these images are "essential to how scientific objects and orderly relationships are revealed and made analyzable."[7] What kinds of relationships are created in the images in *Danforth's*? Part of the answer to this question lies in a close textual investigation of the medium of the image employed. Thus as important as *what* is pictured in *Danforth's* images is *how* these objects are represented. Some of the images found in *Danforth's* are photographic, some are drawn. Why is one mode of representation chosen over another in representing certain anatomical structures? What is more appropriate about photography in one case and drawing in another? How does the choice of drawing or photograph influence the meaning and authority of the representation?

Of the photographs found in *Danforth's*, there is a most glaring and surprising absence. Among the scores of images, there is no photographic representation of healthy, normal genitalia. Where there are numerous black-and-white photographs of pathological external genitalia, as well as black-and-white and color photographs of pathological cervixes, there is not a single reproduction of a healthy cervix or of healthy genitalia.

The words "healthy" and "normal" are used throughout this discussion of textbook images to refer to the wide variety of nonpathological anatomy found on and in healthy bodies. While these terms may be limiting and normalizing, they create a discursive alternative to the largely pathology-oriented medical discourse. This alternative is central to the disciplines of gynecology and obstetrics since its practitioners, unlike many other health care providers, so often encounter well patients in their practices—women simply needing a pap smear or routine prenatal care. For this reason, it is especially important to consider how textbooks present wellness versus illness or abnormality. If only abnormal or pathological anatomy is shown, it must be assumed that practitioners and students understand the wide range of healthy and normal anatomy that exists. I do not mean to imply here that images of healthy genitals are necessarily "positive" representations while images of diseased genitals are inherently "negative." Rather, in identifying representational trends and idiosyncrasies, I am locating the way *Danforth's* communicates notions about the female body. In examining *Danforth's* photographic treatment of female genitals, it becomes clear that the healthy, normal female body in its variety of forms is excluded, whereas abnormal and pathological anatomy is widely represented.

In fact, the very first photograph of external genitalia in *Danforth's* is of ambiguous genitalia. Its caption reads: "Ambiguous external genitalia of a newborn female fetus whose mother inadvertently took a norgesterol-containing oral contraceptive during the first trimester. The infant exhibited clitoral enlargement (A) and persistence of the urogenital sinus (B)" (see Figure 7). While one will never view photographs of normal, healthy female genitalia in *Danforth's*, one is immediately confronted with ambiguity and, further, an ambiguity in need of attention due to the possible psychosocial consequences of an enlarged clitoris (undersized penis). As the textbook notes, "A difficult and potentially psychologically devastating event is the delivery of an infant that is not clearly recognizable as either male or female."[8] The ambiguous, particularly when referring to sex or gender, is akin to the pathological. The medical establishment systematically produces methods for dealing with such ambiguity, so that discrete gender and sex categories may be maintained. Ambiguous genitalia or hermaphroditism pollutes the boundaries that separate the two sexes.[9] This is similar to the way that homosexuality, with its "gender ambiguity," has been pathologized by the medical establishment.[10] The ambiguous and pathological are shown in photographs; the healthy and normal are not.

Among the many photographs of pathological anatomy is Figure 8, captioned "Carcinoma *in situ* in healthy-appearing cervix."[11] Often the caption serves to fix or anchor the image. Here it warns the viewer that the truth is not readily visible;[12] although the cervix may *appear* healthy, it is actually cancerous. Appearances and photographs can be deceptive. The image lies, making the viewer dependent upon the honest caption. The idea that a photograph lies goes against a more prevalent and commonsense way that photographs are understood: as imaging what is "real" by means of the reproductive function of the camera. In the case of the "healthy-appearing" cervix, it is therefore not the photograph that lies so much as the cervix. It is assumed that the photograph represents the cervix accurately; but the cervix does not tell the truth, sporting the appearance of a normal cervix when it is actually pathological. Although *Danforth's* never offers a photograph of a healthy, normal cervix, it presents a photo of a cervix that appears healthy, but in fact is not.

This image of a healthy-appearing cervix is far outnumbered by photographs depicting anatomy very clearly pathological in appearance. Most photographs of genitalia picture gross malformation due to pathology: genitals with huge

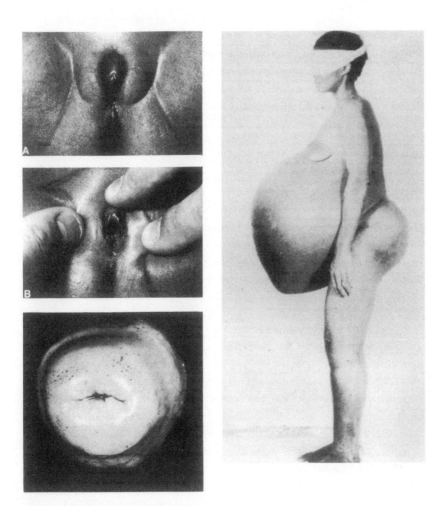

Figure 7. "Ambiguous external
genitalia of a newborn."
Figure 8. "Carcinoma *in situ* in
healthy-appearing cervix."
Figure 9. "Patient with huge benign
cystadenoma of ovary."

growths, prolapses, or lesions. Why are female genitals photographically represented as pathological? One logical answer would be that clinicians need to understand what pathology looks like. But the counterresponse to this would be that, given the very private nature of female genitals, it is as important that clinicians understand what normal, healthy genitals look like. In addition to the profuse number of photographs of pathological vulvas and female bodies, why are we not offered an array of photos of healthy, normal anatomy?

If we consider Freud to be the master informant of (and on) patriarchy's unconscious, we are provided with some possible answers as to why *Danforth's* photographically represents female genitals as pathological. Freud notes that the single most traumatic experience for the male child is viewing female genitalia, out of which arises a lifelong condition known as castration anxiety and an aptitude for engaging in fetishism. In pornography, fetish objects may take the form of stockings, slips, and high-heeled shoes. Is it possible that *pathology* becomes the fetish in the medical context, that it becomes the visible object on which the male physician may concentrate in order to disavow the missing penis? Although female gynecologists are becoming more the norm than the exception, physicians in positions of power, including those editing textbooks, are still predominantly male or positioned as male spectators.

Could this explanation of pathology as fetish also account for the frequent inclusion of images of bodies with extreme manifestations of pathological conditions? For example, one photograph that is used in a number of gyne textbooks including *Danforth's* pictures a woman with a 128-pound ovarian cyst (see Figure 9). She is shown full body, in profile, her belly extraordinarily distended from the residing cyst. A large white blindfold covers the woman's eyes and nose, thus obscuring her identity. This is a curious exception to other photographs in *Danforth's*, in which, as I will discuss later in this chapter, manipulation of the image occurs after it is printed, by cropping so that the head is excluded or by overlaying a rectangular black band over the model's eyes. This postprinting manipulation of the model's eyes inevitably signifies differently than the use of an actual blindfold at the time the photo was taken. In addition, the woman pictured in this photo is of African descent. Was the white blindfold chosen in order to offset her skin color and highlight the masking of her face? The white blindfold carries overtones of enslavement and punishment, pointing backwards historically to J. Marion Sims's gynecological experiments on slaves. There are other ways in which this image is strangely familiar; in an ethnographic visual tradition that commonly depicts "natives" barefoot, naked, and posed in a similar manner, this photograph is reminiscent of images included in such magazines as *National Geographic*. However, the blindfold and the obvious pathology code the image differently. The woman appears as vulnerable both to the pathology and edema (water retention) that bloats her body as well as to the medical establishment that has blindfolded her. But why include this photo at all? If the point of these textbook images is to help clinicians spot pathology, what is the rationale for including an image of a pathology that would be so hard to miss? Does "larger," and therefore more highly visible, pathology better function as fetish? Furthermore, does pathology function as a *comforting* fetish because it absolutely demands medical intervention? Taken to an extreme, pathology on or near female genitalia may also serve as a rationale for the missing penis, a remnant of the illness that *ate* it. Perhaps it is not a lack that is threatening but rather an *excess*. The fact is that even if no pathology exists, there *is* something there— namely, a vulva with labia, a clitoris, and so on, a marginal site occupying both the inside and outside, an abject space (according to Julia Kristeva) that threatens to devour the penis (vagina dentata).[13]

Without turning to a Freudian explanation—so clearly bogged down with problematic and disturbing assumptions—it is still possible to wonder at the photographs included in *Danforth's* and other textbooks and question this fascination with extreme pathology. The display of excess pathology can be linked to the tradition of the circus sideshow. In the sideshow, pathological, anomalous, and often grotesque conditions that would normally remain private are presented for public consumption and titillation. In the medical textbook, as in the sideshow, the display of extreme and grotesque pathology is constructed as clinically exciting and noteworthy, in effect relegating normal anatomy to the realm of the mundane and boring. Such a display of pathology distances the viewer from the spectacle. A polarization occurs between viewer and spectacle; the viewer is assured of his or her normalcy and the freak relegated to the role of aberration.[14] The caption in medical textbooks serves as the barker's pitch, announcing to all who pass by exactly what phenomenon is being presented. However, rather than simply viewing the spectacle for entertainment, the medical textbook viewer is positioned as one who must be able to properly identify and intervene in order to remove or fix such freakishness.

Danforth's viewers are offered two very different pitches: the "healthy-appearing cervix" image and caption alert the viewers to the fact that healthy-appearing anatomy can be deceptive, while the images of obvious and extreme pathology with their accompanying captions reassure the viewer of the readability of the pathological body. What they have in common is that both cases present anatomy in need of medical intervention. Excluded from *Danforth's* is the image with accompanying pitch that would announce anatomy that is normal and healthy and therefore *not* in need of medical intervention.

The only set of photographs in *Danforth's* that shows a healthy vulva is used to serve a different purpose: captioned "Spontaneous delivery" (Figure 10), this twelve-frame series shows a white woman giving birth. The photo includes the knees, legs, drape sheet, and genitals of the birthing woman in lithotomy position, heels in footrests, knees open. The photos are cropped in such a way that her face, eyes, hands, arms, and so forth are not included. The hands of the physician are introduced in the very first frame as they perform a midline episiotomy (a cut with scissors in order to "widen" the vaginal opening) on the woman's shaved vulva. The assumption that an episiotomy is necessarily part of a spontaneous delivery is curious given that many childbirth educators, midwives, and physicians consider it, in many cases, an unnecessary and unhelpful medical intervention, opting instead for perineal massage and possible tears.[15] Likewise, some practitioners, particularly midwives, maintain that shaving pubic hair during labor can actually be harmful, considering it to be an "unjustified assault."[16] However, the only image of normal delivery in this textbook depicts an episiotomy and shaved vulva at its start, as though they were a necessary and integral part of any delivery.

Similarly, the series of photographs of this delivery begins documentation at the point that medical intervention begins, supporting the idea, prevalent since the rise of obstetrics as a discipline, that birth is an inherently pathological occurrence and therefore an "occasion for medical surveillance and treatment."[17] The series does not start with the beginning of labor, rather the delivery begins with the intervening hands of the physician. Likewise, the woman assumes a passive birthing position. No alternatives are pictured such as upright positions that include standing, squatting, or crouching. Although we are told by the caption that this is a *spontaneous* delivery, the photographs' narrative offers a different picture. The woman's contribution to the birth as represented in the photographs is minimal. In this series, it appears as if the process of birthing is something that is enacted upon the reclining woman pictured: there is no evidence of her active participation; the physician appears to be doing all the work. Although these photographs are the only occasion in *Danforth's* in which a healthy, normal vulva is shown, the vulva has already been shaved and is first pictured as it undergoes transformation at the hands of the physician, hands that remain in the frame until the end of the successful "spontaneous delivery."[18]

Because of the mechanical recording function of the camera, photographs are commonly assumed to simply present reality.[19] The fashioning of the photograph—its framing, the lighting, and so on—is made transparent, particularly in a scientific context where photos are provided as visual evidence of scientific truths. However, while photographs may reference the real, they are not mi-

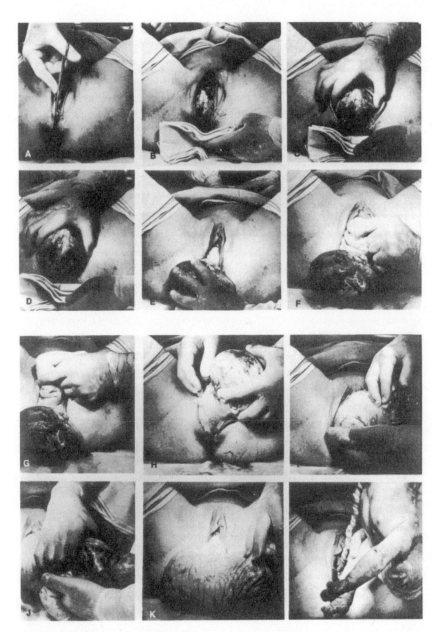

Figure 10. "Spontaneous delivery."

metic representations. The "real" that is continuously constructed by *Danforth's* is that vulvas and cervixes are diseased and that a spontaneous delivery demands medical intervention.

Certainly one would think that not every obstetrics and gynecology textbook excludes photographs of healthy, normal genitalia. Indeed there are limitations to close readings of single texts as they may not necessarily reflect the variation found among medical textbooks themselves. And yet, in the medical textbooks I examined aside from *Danforth's*, I found little variety. In fact, I discovered only one instance of a photograph of healthy, normal female genitalia—an unobscured color photograph in a photographic gross anatomy atlas.[20] The entire atlas is comprised of labeled color photographs of sectioned, dissected corpses. But the photograph of unobscured, labeled genitals looks remarkably alive, unlike any other photograph in the book. The tissue is moist and pink, rather than the dried, miscolored anatomy pictured in the rest of the images. Also, the vulva in this photograph is intact; there is no evidence of dissection as there is in the photographs of sectioned parts. No caption distinguishes this photo as living female genitalia, and it is surrounded by photographs on the same page that undeniably picture corpses. Is the reader to be fooled into believing that these normal genitalia are dead? If the reader does recognize this photograph as a living exception (and the only one in the entire textbook), how does this code female genitalia? By placing an image of living genitals in the context of dead female genitals, is the potential pornographics of living genitalia displaced? Is the pornographic quality heightened by a sort of necrophilia? Does this juxtaposition of living with dead genitals reflect some anxiety regarding birth (the vulva as birthing exit) and death (what is the afterlife of genitals)? In discussing the circus sideshow, Susan Stewart explains that, alive or dead, the freak is still both a freak and a valuable spectacle. She offers the example of John Hunter, the father of British surgery, who "was just as happy to have the bones of the giant James Byrne as to study him alive."[21] Is the vulva as an object of clinical study the same, living or dead?

Photography as a medium has long been associated with death. Photographic images cessate life the moment the shutter clicks. In his book *Camera Lucida*, Roland Barthes discusses the photograph as "this image which produces Death while trying to preserve life."[22] Since photographs already signify death in some way, photographs of sectioned corpses are an interesting semiotic doubling. The photograph of living external genitalia found in a gross anatomy atlas may be an attempt to "preserve life," but because it is a photograph and a photograph placed in the context of sectioned corpses, it simultaneously "produces Death." Given its surroundings, this photograph of genitalia may actually signify the *living dead*, a haunting and haunted spectacle. Regardless of how it is read, this image of a lone vulva in the land of the dead is a glaring exception to the rule that photographs—particularly color photos—of healthy (perhaps alluring) female genitalia will not appear in medical textbooks.

Although there are no photographs that feature healthy, normal female genitalia in *Danforth's*, there are two photographic sequences that do focus on healthy, living female bodies. Both present standards of development, the first focusing on breast development and the second on pubic hair development. Figure 11 is captioned "Standards for evaluating breast development"; it shows a series of five numbered photographs of a specific woman's breasts as they progress from preadolescence through adulthood. In the sequence entitled "Standards for evaluating pubic hair development" (Figure 12), the pubic area is treated in much the same way: sectioned from hip to mid-thigh and numbered sequentially according to the development of the female, who is standing with legs together.[23] While growth may be the subject of these photographic series, there are once again overtones of death. The way the photos are cropped make the sectioned women, particularly the breast model, look like decapitated corpses. These photos that document the growth of individual body parts might fall somewhere between the photographic and the cinematic. André Bazin notes that a photograph "embalms time" and "the cinema is objectivity in time."[24] The temporal progression of these photographic series references the filmic; still frames mark growth with time similarly to fast-motion studies of a budding sprout.[25] In addition the photographs charting breast development remarkably resemble mug shots: the upright female is shown front view and then to her side. However, unlike mug shots, these photographs are cropped in such a way as to exclude the woman's face. This exclusion is most likely an attempt to protect the woman's anonymity and modesty by removing her most public feature. Whereas criminal mug shots concentrate on the face, the primary site through which an individual may be identified (no two faces are alike), these breast shots are presented as the absolute standard of development (all breasts grow alike). Even though breasts and genitals are features as unique and distinctive as faces, the fact that they are normally covered leads to the understanding that as long as the woman's face is hidden her breasts or genitals will not be recognized.

There could be another reason for excluding the woman's face. By cropping the photographs so that only pertinent body parts are shown, the woman is appropriately sectioned for scientific study, as object for the medical gaze. Here, cropping the photograph serves the same function as the drape sheet in the classic pelvic exam scenario: it sections the woman for examination, placing her eyes, face, and mouth backstage. If the woman's eyes had been included in these photographs, their presence might have evoked a different and more suggestive

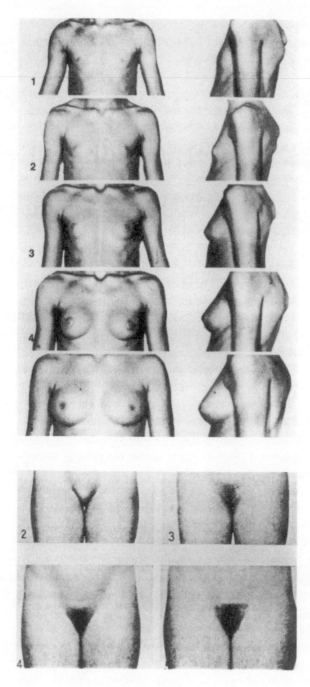

Figure 11. "Standards
for evaluating breast
development."
Figure 12. "Standards
for evaluating pubic
hair development."

meaning. As Annette Kuhn notes: "In offering itself as both spectacle and truth, the photograph suggests that the woman in the picture, rather than the image itself, is responsible for soliciting the spectator's gaze."[26] This solicitation is often coded as suggestive or even pornographic. In order to maintain the "maximum authority" that *Danforth's* requires, female volition—a volition that might point to the pleasure of being looked at—must be policed. If the woman's eyes were included in the photographs' frames, questions of pleasure and desire with regard to both the photographed model and the clinician or medical student viewer could "enter the picture."

The woman's head and face are cropped or, in some cases, her eyes are banded, reducing the woman to a passive object of the gaze, devoid of identity and missing the potential for pleasure or desire. And yet, banding the anonymous woman's eyes may also function differently. Blindfolds and postproduction banding have been used by pornographers as a way of making their objects less human, "to make him or her into 'only' a body."[27] When the object of the gaze has banded eyes, the subject position of the viewer is potentially more powerful. The viewer observing the photograph, by definition, *can see* the photo, whereas the woman pictured *cannot see*. Thus there is a potential sadistic erotics implicit in this voyeuristic subject position.[28] Notions of criminality (e.g., mug shots) and victimization (e.g., banded eyes) collapse in these photographic representations of women, policing the portrayal of those parts of the female body (breast and pubic areas) that reference female sexuality by employing the ever-popular motifs of excessive villain and passive prey.

These few views of healthy female anatomy markedly contrast the overwhelming number of photographic representations of pathological female bodies. However, an individual's breast or pubic area is offered as a normal standard, disregarding the immense variation of breast and pubic area development found in normal, healthy women. If a woman has breasts or a body that is differently sized or shaped than those of the women pictured, does this mean that she is "below standard"? Furthermore, how were these women picked as *standard*? Why were thin bodies chosen as standard? What are the implications of choosing two white bodies as standard? Why wasn't the body of a woman of color or of a large woman chosen as standard? As discussed in chapter 2, the choice of whiteness as standard plays into an extensive history of constructing whiteness as normal and people of color as pathological.

In his historical analysis of the constructions of the normal and the pathological, Georges Canguilhem surmises that "the concepts of norm and average must be considered as two different concepts: it seems vain to try to reduce them to one by wiping out the originality of the first."[29] The photographs, which are pre-

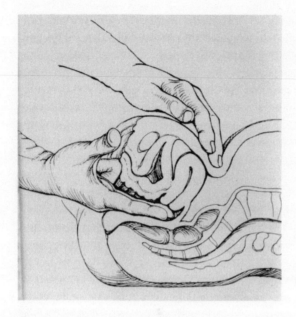

Figure 13. "Bimanual
examination, *first step*."

sented as standards for evaluating female body parts, disregard the "originality"
and multiformity of that which is normal by replacing it with an arbitrary, limiting, and racially specific average. These breast and pubic hair standards are as
arbitrary and limiting as ideals regarding female beauty upheld by popular magazines and other mainstream media in which perfect bodily proportion is discussed at length. Articles regarding ideal thigh and upper arm widths, eyebrow
shape and location, and feminine musculature are pictorially endorsed by
models chosen for their adherence to such beauty ideals. Once again, features
commonly associated with whiteness are regularly upheld as important standards (e.g., straight hair, thin noses, etc.). These standards for self-evaluation are
not unlike those photographic standards of breast and pubic hair development
against which clinicians are to measure patients. However, in the case of beauty
magazines the viewer has a greater chance of understanding that such standards
are the result of current fashions, while in medical textbooks such standards
carry the authority and universality of scientific inquiry.

Diagram

Where a photo is often seen as a simple recording of the real, a drawn image is
recognized as a transformation from the real, a transformation that divides the
"significant from the insignificant."[30] In scientific imaging, the drawing or dia-

gram is an idealized rendering. Diagrams in *Danforth's* serve to *clarify* the female reproductive apparatus, rendering anatomical structures that might be too difficult to clearly visualize by photographic means. As Michael Lynch argues in discussing scientific representation, "*relative to the photograph*, the diagram is an *eidetic* image and not merely a simplified image."[31] The drawings, accompanied by their labels, create an orderly hyperreal, a real better than reality, in many ways viewed as more accurate than the photograph. For instance, the drawing entitled "Bimanual examination, *first step*" (Figure 13) shows a cross-sectioned female body with the physician's fingers already in place. The diagrammatic medium allows for a visualization of what is usually invisible: the physician's hand inside the patient and its relation to female internal structures. The drawing represents an impossible perspective, an unnatural cross section, a popular visualizing perspective in wildlife documentaries reminiscent of the terrarium view of an ant farm or other animal's burrow. Employing crafty diagrammatic rendering, science triumphs over nature's fascinating holes and canals, making visible the secret home of the ant or the mysterious internal genitalia.[32] In this sense, the medical diagram has more in common with imaginary visions of high art than the documentarity of photography.

The set of drawings entitled "Hirsutism from 1 (mild hirsutism) to 4 (severe hirsutism) in nine areas" (Figure 14) works similarly to the series of photographs of the standard development of breasts and pubic area. Like those photographs, this drawing serves to normalize on a numeric scale. Why choose a diagrammatic rather than photographic mode of representation? Given that hirsutism does not occur to all degrees on a single individual, it is not as easy to standardize photographically as breast or pubic hair development. Medical photographers would have to find ideal levels of hirsutism in a variety of people and place them side by side. However, there could be another reason. The fact that hirsutism occurs on a woman's face could make the diagram more fitting than the photograph given the emphasis on maintaining the model's anonymity. The rendered faces in this diagram, however, are still featureless. It is important to recognize that this normalizing diagram, like the previous standardizing photographs of the breast and pubic area, associates whiteness with standards. The drawn model has typically white features such as straight, shoulder-length hair. As in the breast and pubic hair development photos, whiteness is presented as the norm.[33]

"Perineum of the female" (Figure 15) is the first view of female genitalia in *Danforth's*. The artist of the diagram alters the perspective of female anatomy to such a degree that one must orient oneself with the provided labels in order to understand that it is female genitals that are in fact being represented. No drawn legs, buttocks, pubic hair, or abdomen accompany the perineum.[34] Is there con-

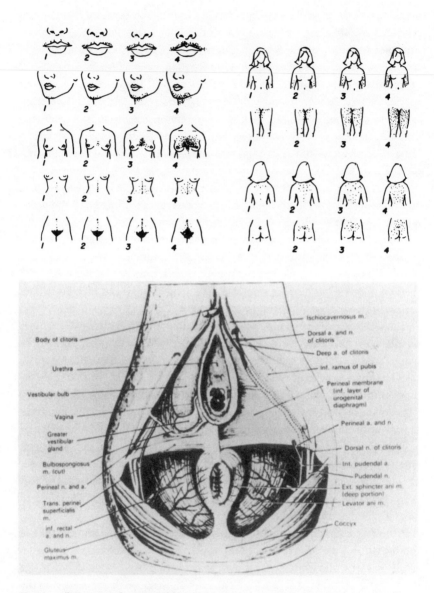

Figure 14. "Hirsutism from 1 (mild hirsutism) to 4 (severe hirsutism) in nine areas."
Figure 15. "Perineum of the female."

cern that if these (unnecessary?) contextualizing attachments were included this diagram could threaten the boundaries of pornographic illustration? Are images of genitalia so pornographically problematic that diagrams of normal genitalia exclude any remnants of recognizable bodily accompaniment even at the expense of the accuracy of the diagram? Not every medical specialty employs such obscurity. On the second page of a commonly used ophthalmology textbook a large photograph of an eye is presented.[35] A healthy eye is shown photographed, healthy female genitalia are not. Diagrams in *Danforth's* normalize the female body, operating similarly to the photo sequences that document standard breast and pubic development. A theoretical rendering of assumedly normal, healthy genitalia is presented in lieu of photographs of the variety of forms that normal, healthy genitalia take. In *Danforth's* an overwhelming consistency emerges: Normalized female genitalia are drawn and pathological female genitalia are photographed. It becomes apparent that female bodies in *Danforth's* must be coded in particular ways for proper public presentation.

The Penis

Does the construction of the male body in medical textbooks operate in a different way from that of the female body? Are male genitalia subject to the same systems of representation? *General Urology* is equivalent to *Danforth's* in that it too is a one-volume overview commonly used by medical schools.[36] In *General Urology* there are *no* close-up photographs of a penis. There are many MRI, CT scan, sonogram, and radionuclide images, so it is clear that the editors or publishers were not simply trying to cut costs by excluding photographic representations. However, even in the chapter titled "Skin Diseases of the External Genitalia" there are no photographs of the conditions discussed. Likewise, in the chapter on sexually transmitted diseases, there is not a single visual reference to pathological genitalia even though visualizable symptoms such as warts, herpes lesions, and chancroids are discussed.[37]

Pathology and the penis are left photographically unrepresented. If what is photographed is coded as "real," what is the significance of presenting photographs of only diseased vulvas in gynecology textbooks and no photographs whatsoever of penises in urology textbooks? While written about, the pathologized penis is not represented visually, nor is the penis fixed as pathological in the same way that the vulva is. In addition, a photo of the penis, healthy or not, would secure a referent, limiting the penis in its photographic materiality. Photos would also fix penis size, not allowing for the normal variation that might be reassuring to certain viewers. For instance, would there ever be a series of images titled "Standards for evaluating penis development" in line with those focusing on breast and pubic hair development?

There was a two-photograph series in *General Urology* that did present bodily outsides. The first photo pictured an individual with Klinefelter's syndrome standing against a height chart. The photo next to this one presented the same man's undersized testes undergoing measurement. Klinefelter's syndrome is a genetic condition in which the individual is born with an extra X chromosome, resulting in some feminization and small testes and penis. In *General Urology* the only photographs of male genitalia are those of an individual who does not qualify as a "real man." In fact, the evidence of this individual's pathology is his feminization and his measurably undersized testes. A penis belonging to a genetically normal male, diseased or not, is never shown in a photograph.

Western medical textbooks, including urology textbooks, have been created by and for a predominantly male medical audience. Due to deep-seated homophobia, there is a great deal of anxiety regarding men's viewing other men's genitals. Ironically, the spectacle of an erect penis ejaculating or a "money shot" is a prevalent trope in mainstream pornographic film.[38] Excluding photographs of penises in *General Urology* eliminates the possibility of homoerotic or pornographic viewing. Furthermore, because images of pathological penises have been excluded from *General Urology*, the viewer is prevented from identifying with the man whose penis is diseased; if such images were included, they might prevent the viewer from achieving proper clinical distance from the object of study. Whereas diseased vulvas and other female body parts with large pathology are the clinical fetishes in the context of *Danforth's*, there is no parallel fetish in the case of *General Urology*.

There are a fair number of drawings in *General Urology*, almost none of which represent the outside of the penis. Indeed, to take it to an absurd extreme, if aliens were to look to *General Urology* for information on normal human anatomy, they might think that there is no skin covering the penis at all.[39] Drawings of the penis serve to normalize and generalize it in its *healthy* state. While female genitalia are also drawn in order to normalize and generalize them, there is such a profusion of photographs of diseased cervixes and vulvas that this abundance of images may serve to "fix" the female as *pathological*.

Apparently Female

One set of photographic images in *Danforth's* is reminiscent of the "healthy-appearing cervix" image, and it is one of the few instances in which there is a full frontal image of an uncropped woman. The beginning of the caption reads, "Androgen insensitivity in 18-year-old apparent female with primary amenor-

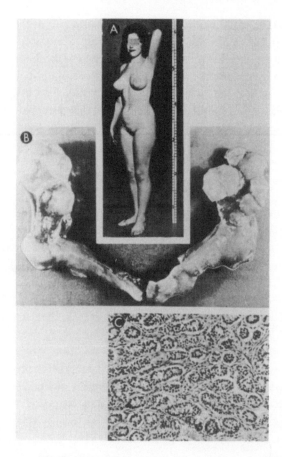

Figure 16. "Androgen insensitivity in 18-year-old apparent female."

rhea, minimal sexual hair, large breasts and areolae, but small nipples" (Figure 16).[40] On first glance, we may identify the individual pictured as a woman, but the caption assures the reader that she is an "apparent female," questioning her gender-sex status while simultaneously invoking it. Once again, gender-sex ambiguities signify a pathological danger requiring medical attention while the caption informs us that the body lies by appearing to be something it is not. A band is placed over the apparent female's eyes to obscure her face, in the manner discussed earlier. The photograph of the woman is situated above another photograph that pictures her surgically removed "Gonads and rudimentary uterine structures." The arrangement of these two photographs makes it seem as though the "apparent female" is surrounded by her insufficient reproductive structures. Photomicrographs of these structures (photographs of what can be seen when looking under a microscope) are located beneath the two photographs. The organization of these three photographs situates the most magnified part at the base, leaving the least magnified image of the woman at the top. The photographs lead the viewer from the top photo of the "apparent" female to the foundational photomicrographs; from top to bottom, from skin surface to magnified cells, the images seem to zoom into the basic biological *truth*. Like a deductive sleuth, the grouping of images tells a story. It becomes apparent that the apparent female is not what she appears. Here genitalia are no longer authentic sex or gender markers. It is necessary to go further, past the privates to the more private microscopic world of cellular certainty. At this infinitesimal level the telling evidence is found. The caption reads: "Note marked resemblance to fetal testis." Appearances may be tricky.

Scale is a sort of carnivalesque joke in this set of images. The "apparent female" stands next to a ruler to indicate her height and yet she is surrounded by her own blown-up internal parts. Her gonads and uterine structures look like mammoth dinosaur bones in relation to her body. These photographs are coded as medical: a pathological body with an obscured face, a black-and-white photo, flat lighting, a caption explaining the pathology. And yet, if the caption were ignored, this set of images could slip into the realm of the pornographic. The juxtaposition of these three photos creates a narrative, a thrilling erotic story about a blindfolded, naked woman who finds herself trapped by her own, now gigantic (un)reproductive parts. Constructed like a dadaist collage, this set of images might slip into the category of "art." Ironically, the "apparent female" is also distinctly reminiscent of the classic nineteenth-century nude in body shape and in suppression of pubic and axillary (armpit) hair. But her large breasts, lack of pu-

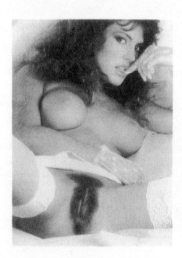
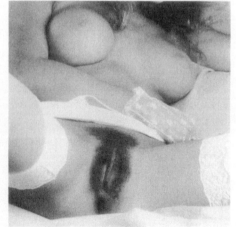

bic and axillary hair, and classic cheesecake pose (hand behind the head) are also characteristic of specific genres of mainstream pornography.[41]

One reason this image of a whole naked female body is allowable in a medical textbook may be her "fortuitous" pathological condition of hairlessness. Does the erasure of pubic hair, a disappearance so precious to classical painting, aid the viewer in subscribing to a lack of any female genitals whatsoever? Conversely, the presence of pubic hair would therefore signify the presence of genitalia. If this were the case, the "apparent female" may safely be photographed due to her smooth surface. However, porn mags such as *Shaved* court hairlessness, making the "apparent female" a viable candidate. A lack of pubic hair in the pornographic context might serve a number of functions—referencing youthfulness while permitting an unobscured visualization of the genitals. Pubic and axillary hair (or the lack thereof) produce a multiplicity of cultural meanings, signifying differently within and between the categories of art, pornography, and medicine.

In examining images found in *Danforth's* I have questioned whether medical photos disavow or allow for pornographic possibilities. Can the opposite be true as well? Can the medical be present in a pornographic image? Figure 17 is a "beaver" shot from *Penthouse*.[42] This full-page photo is part of a series entitled "Beauty and the Beast," a piece that offers a short, erotic bio of this twenty-four-year-old model-actress and her horror film roles.[43] The model enacts the soliciting gaze, a decidedly pornographic look and one that is carefully regulated in gynecological textbooks. If the model's face and head are cropped, enlisting a

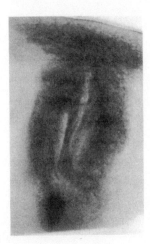

Figure 17. Beauty and the Beast.
Figures 18 and 19. Beauty and the
Beast (cropped).

common medical textbook image method, the possibility of assigning her the agency of a look is eliminated, but vestiges of clothing still remain (see Figure 18). Clothing is entirely absent in gynecological textbook images. In pornography, clothing may signify the ability to undress or strip. In medical practice in the United States, the patient undresses without the physician present. Costumed in gown and drape for proper medicalization, the patient is both disassociated from her clothes and daily identity and prepared for segmented examination. By ridding the gynecological scenario of clothing entirely, the sexually charged appearance of partial dress is disavowed. In the porn photo, the stockings, gloves, and slip alert the reader to the fact that this is a pornographic image. If we crop the photo again to exclude all vestiges of clothing and accessories, all that remains of the original image is a color close-up of healthy genitals (see Figure 19). Can this image be coded as either pornographic or medical? It is reminiscent of the color image of genitals found in the photographic atlas containing mostly representations of corpses, however it is not surrounded by images of dissected bodies. While fairly clinical, this photo would indeed be a rarity in a medical textbook, since it shows a healthy, normal vulva in no particular need of medical intervention. But this photo would also be a rarity in a pornographic context. Whereas female sexuality, desire, desirability, and the soliciting look are denied in gynecological images, they are the basic elements of pornographic images. Without appropriate accoutrements, this stark image of healthy, normal female genitalia would be a very strange find in a pornographic context.[44] Both the medical and the pornographic scenarios require the proper dressing, be it pathology or lace, to create the proper mise-en-scène or narrative context for the exposed vulva.[45]

Making a Spectacle in/out of Yourself

This hypothetical color image of healthy genitals could be one of a series of photos found in a self-help medical book published by the Federation of Feminist Women's Health Centers, aptly titled *New View of a Woman's Body* (*NVWB*).[46] The only photographs in *NVWB* are full-page assortments of color close-up images: one page of healthy external genitalia and one of cervixes (see Figure 20). Each image is accompanied by a lengthy caption that attempts to situate the part pictured. For example, the text accompanying the top right image of a cervix reads, "This woman's cervix has a few small red blotches near the os and you can see a clear mucus secretion coming out. Her vaginal wall, right next to the cervix, has a ripply texture. She is six weeks pregnant." This caption is different from those in *Danforth's*, which name only the object present in the image with-

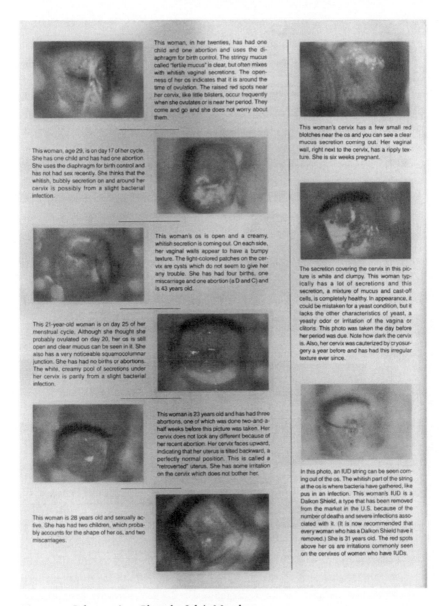

Figure 20. Color cervixes. Photo by Sylvia Morales.

out reference to an accompanying woman. The caption at the top of the first page of external genitalia prefaces the photographs: "This series of photos of the vulva and clitoris shows some of the many healthy, normal variations of the size, shape, color and texture of the features of the clitoris." In direct contradiction to medical texts such as *Danforth's*, *NVWB* offers a selection of photos of healthy, normal anatomy. Heeding Canguilhem's warning, the authors of *NVWB* attempt to present the originality of that which is normal, instead of replacing it with a sole image that would serve as an arbitrary and limiting average.

Both *Danforth's* and *NVWB* use the medium of photography to clearly present what is considered unique or specific. In *Danforth's*, the specificity of the pathological demands the photographic medium. Emphasis is placed on the number of possible pathological manifestations and the importance of recognizing them in their individuality. In *NVWB* the uniqueness of normal anatomical variation demands the photographic medium. If presented to medical students, color photographs of a variety of women's genitals would offer them a nuanced sense of anatomical difference, a view otherwise difficult to obtain in print given the systematic privatization of female genitals. An understanding of normality fosters an understanding of what is abnormal. Without an understanding of normal variation, every change in texture or shape may be mistaken for a pathology.

In line with Luce Irigaray's notion that women have multiple sexual organs, the women who wrote *NVWB* redefine the clitoral area—a key player in female sexual pleasure—so that the term includes a much larger proportion of the genitals.[47] This move is an attempt to bring female sexuality, desire, and pleasure to the center of women's health discourse. And indeed such discourse is missing in *Danforth's*. Whereas *General Urology* includes a chapter titled "Physiology of Erection and Pathophysiology of Impotence," *Danforth's* devotes virtually no space to a discussion of the mechanics of female sexual response or the possibility of the lack thereof. In *NVWB* however, a chapter entitled "The Clitoris: A Feminist Perspective" provides drawings of clitoral self-exam (see Figure 21) and of the various phases of clitoral excitement, with women touching their vulvas and spreading their own labia for clear visualization. It even presents diagrams that compare the clitoris to the penis and vice versa with regard to unaroused and erect states (demarcated using dotted lines). *NVWB*'s creators have a clear agenda in maintaining that both men and women have physiological responses to sexual arousal, a fact almost entirely overlooked by *Danforth's* but addressed with an entire chapter in *General Urology*.

In both photographs and drawings in *NVWB*, women are pictured touching and observing their own vulvas. Although *Danforth's* provides a diagram of a

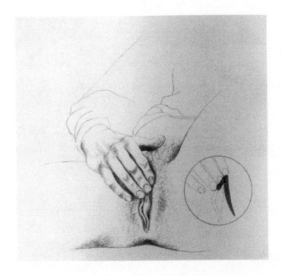

Figure 21. "A woman
doing self-examination of
the clitoris." Illustration
by Suzann Gage.

woman engaging in a self-breast-exam, no woman, drawn or photographed, is
clearly shown touching her genitals, nor are there any images connected with female orgasm or sexual response. Rather it is the practitioner who touches the
woman's vulva in images such as "spontaneous delivery," with the woman's
hands nowhere in sight. Except for self-breast-exam, there is no presentation of
self-touch in *Danforth's* as a possible or beneficial practice (despite the fact that
more and more practitioners advocate vulvar self-exam). In *NVWB* self-touch
is consistently represented, but mostly in diagram. Photos of women touching
themselves are cropped so that only fingers and revealed vulva are shown. Is it
possible that, in both texts, photos of women touching themselves were pur-
posely avoided in order to avoid referencing mainstream pornography, where
masturbation is so often a theme?

    As discussed earlier in this chapter, another common pornographic trope, the
soliciting gaze of the model, is completely avoided in *Danforth's* through techniques such as blindfolding, banding, and cropping. However, in *NVWB*
women are shown both meeting the spectator's gaze and observing their own
anatomy. Once again, however, this occurs solely in diagrammatic form. Their
drawn faces exhibit expressions signifying self-observation and concentration
rather than the expressionless, manipulated faces of the women shown in *Danforth's*. These images are reflective of the process the illustrator, Suzann Gage,
went through in order to create them. In the introduction to *NVWB* the writers
describe the way Gage and the models, most of whom were experienced "self-
helpers," conferred on the best way to portray a particular idea. The model then

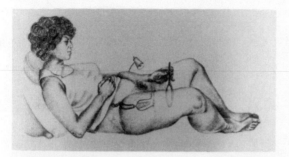

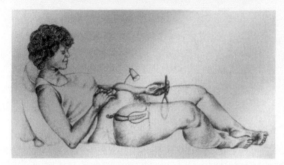

Figure 22. "A woman
doing self-examination."
Illustration by
Suzann Gage.

gave herself a vaginal self-exam and Gage would follow with an exam to determine the model's uterine size, location, and position. (In the scope of *Danforth's*,
I find it difficult to imagine a non physician illustrator doing a pelvic exam on a
model in order to better understand the intended diagram.) The introduction
goes on to describe the fact that Gage's drawings are based on her studies of English, German, French, and Italian anatomy texts, but that, "still, she has had to
infer much, particularly in her drawings of the clitoris, since an extensive study
of many anatomy and sex education books revealed no cross section of the clitoris." Similarly, the process of the photographer, Sylvia Morales, is described. The
hundreds of photographs she took of cervixes, vulvas, clitorises, and hair patterns, the way she coded photographs with the model's name and medical history, and her extensive experimentation with various lenses and lighting are discussed. This foregrounding of the imaging philosophy and methods used in
NVWB would be impossible in a text like *Danforth's*, given the fact that such a
variety of images—chronologically, authorially, processually, and so on—are
used. Attention in *Danforth's* is not placed on the *construction* or authorship of
these images; rather they are left to "speak for themselves" as inevitable and
truthful reproductions.

Whereas the "standard" that *Danforth's* proposes in photographic series like

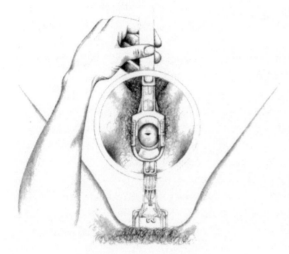

Figure 23. "A view of the
cervix in a mirror."
Illustration by
Suzann Gage.

those that display breast and pubic hair development is that of whiteness and
thinness, in *NVWB*, women of different ethnicities and body shapes are de-
picted. And, unlike *Danforth's*, such differences are included in diagrams. Every
effort is made to maintain the pictured woman's individuality, rather than eras-
ing difference in order to produce a normative standard. Most often, the model's
face and its distinguishing features are shown. No attempt is made to maintain
her anonymity. (However, faces are only pictured in diagrams, not photographs.) The models are not costumed for proper medical consumption with
drape sheets; instead, women are shown partially dressed. In the drawing captioned "A woman doing self-examination," a woman manipulates a medical instrument, taking an active role in her own examination (Figure 22). "A view of
the cervix in a mirror" (Figure 23) offers spectators the perspective of a woman
who engages in cervical self-exam. This spectatorial identification with the
woman who is both model and examiner is a perspective impossible within the
scope of *Danforth's*, where the constructed "real" is that of a pathological female
body requiring medical intervention. In *NVWB*, female anatomy is not so easily
"fixed." It is presented as variable, normally healthy, subject to self-exam and
possibly even self-management.

Not that *NVWB* is the best possible solution. If *Danforth's* codes the vulva as
pathological, *NVWB* leaves us with a pristine vulva. Photographs in *NVWB*
only picture normal, healthy anatomy. Diseased vulvas and cervixes are exclu-

sively drawn, working in converse of the photographed pathology and drawn normalcy of medical textbooks such as *Danforth's*. Why exclude photographs of diseased vulvas? Most likely, the authors of *NVWB* are consciously situating themselves in opposition to texts like *Danforth's* that overemphasize pathology at the expense of acknowledging the variation of normal anatomy. But what is at stake in presenting photos only of healthy anatomy? In excluding photos of diseased genitalia, do authors reproduce the fear of what it might be like to "really find" lesions or warts? In this noticeable absence (as noticeable as the absence of photos of *healthy* genitals in *Danforth's*), does *NVWB* reinforce simplistic notions that would connect the presentation of photos of diseased vulvas with both female victimization and promiscuity? Though *NVWB* is clearly constructed in reaction to texts like *Danforth's*, it risks playing into similar binarisms. Whereas *Danforth's* privileges pathology, *NVWB*'s exclusion of photographic representations of pathology could support constructions that ally diseased women with disempowerment and well women with empowerment. The media of drawing and photography bring specific connotations to the ideological construction of the female body when exclusively aligned with either pathology or normalcy.

Afterthoughts

My readings of *Danforth's* images have been unsympathetic, to some degree, to the editors' stated "need" to create a "complete" and "concise" gynecological textbook. For the most part, I have read the images out of their intended context; I have not examined them for their medical exactitude or usefulness, but for their semiotic value in the coding of the category "female." Although such textbooks are seen as practical and helpful and as simply "fitting in" to the largely pathology-based medical institution, I want to assert that these images are neither transparent nor inevitable.[48] The fact that *Danforth's* is a scientific textbook propagates the notion that medical students and physicians are somehow desensitized to textual treatments of bodies and thus read images differently than a lay person such as myself. But the assumption that these trained experts are able to read past such images to the "truth" is a false one. The acquisition of medical knowledge does not somehow exempt medical students or practitioners from the effects of visual ideology, ideology that constructs the categories of female and male in particular ways. Representational practices in turn affect medical practice, and textbook images clearly help structure attitudes, relationships, and other aspects of actual medical practice.

    NVWB is certainly a step in the right direction with its emphasis on self-spectatorship, self-management, female sexual pleasure, and anatomical variety. However, its representational practices risk containment within the same simplistic binaristic logic that limits *Danforth's*. Both works place judgments and values onto conditions of wellness and illness. In creating and using texts, both alternative feminist health advocates and medical practitioners are involved in organizing knowledge about female bodies. Administering health care requires such organization. But a strong analysis of the consequences of various ways of organizing visual, written, and tactile information should be made a central part of medical pedagogy.[49] Likewise, it is essential that those subject to medical intervention as well as self-management (patients and lay people) have the critical tools to decipher representational strategies. What I am advocating is a broader spectrum of types of women's health care texts and a greater variety of readers of those texts. Ideally, medical students should be exposed to *NVWB* and gynecological patients should have the opportunity to consider how texts like *Danforth's* affect the way their bodies are seen and treated.

When leafing through *Danforth's*, I visit a hardbound freak show. I am not titillated, but incredibly disturbed—by the images already discussed but also by diagrams of a hysterectomy found on *page 8*.[50] Within the first ten pages, the potential gynecological practitioner is already being taught how to remove the dangerous, hysteria-inducing organ. Would drawings of techniques for testicular removal or male castration be entertained in the first ten pages of a companion volume? If violence, the sectioning of the female body, and explicit imagery are commonly defining qualities of mainstream pornography, as antiporn, procensorship subscribers insist, images in *Danforth's* may inconspicuously fall into this category. In antiporn terms the public space of the medical textbook *is* dangerous for the female body. Thus if these pro-censorship subscribers were to broaden their perspective, they might want to shift their attention from pornographic texts to medical texts like *Danforth's*.

However, *I* am not proposing that *Danforth's* be taken out of circulation. In fact I think *Danforth's* should be distributed to all women. It should be taught in humanities classrooms, shelved at public libraries throughout the United States, demonstrated door-to-door with critical annotation, and mulled over at ladies' book groups. Maybe *Danforth's* could thus be put to good use as a woman's handbook, a sort of "how they view you" journal. Thus, the freak and the viewer could become one and the same, mending the age-old schism between the aberrant object and the entertained onlooker.

I have these fantasies as I pass *Danforth's* to the attendant who works the medical library reserve shelves. I wonder who will check the book out after me. Will it be a medical student I met while teaching? a medical student who found it impossible to look into my eyes because they were not banded or blindfolded?

5 Retooling the Speculum:
Annie Sprinkle's "Public Cervix Announcement"

To claim that sex is already gendered, already constructed, is not yet to explain in which way the "materiality" of sex is forcibly produced. —Judith Butler, *Bodies That Matter*

It is October 1991. Performance artist, porn star, photographer, and prostitution rights activist Annie Sprinkle is on stage at a small, alternative theater in Chicago. Just before intermission during her traveling one-woman show, "Post Post Porn Modernist: Still in Search of the Ultimate Sexual Experience," Sprinkle begins the "Public Cervix Announcement" (PCA). She presents the audience with two large, oval-shaped, colored drawings: one a cartoonish rendering of the female reproductive organs (cervix, uterus, fallopian tubes, and ovaries), the other a bubblegum pink drawing of what some members of the audience are about to see: a large, round cervix with a dark dot in the middle (the os) (see Figure 24). Sprinkle asks the audience to repeat the anatomical names after her sing-songy phonetical instruction: "you-ter-us, fah-low-pee-an-toobs." Having just performed in Germany, she also has the audience say "uterus" in German. Discarding her drawings, she walks over to the toilette area of her salon set and douches with a long rubber hose; feigning surprise, she giggles as she pees into the porcelain pot (see Figure 25).

Sitting on a chair center stage, Sprinkle offers four reasons for the PCA:

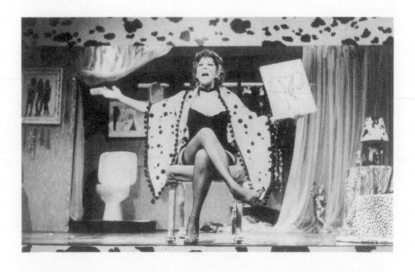

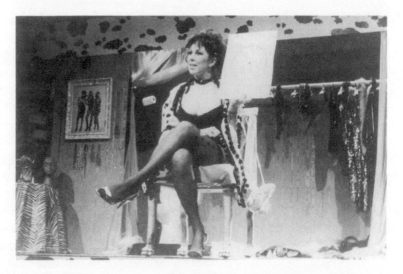

Figure 24. Sprinkle presenting drawings of the female reproductive organs (above) and cervix (below).

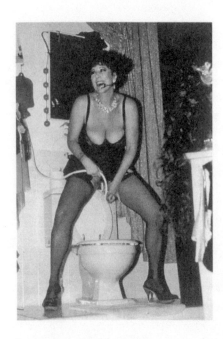

Figure 25. Sprinkle douching
in preparation for the "Public
Cervix Announcement."
Photo by Leslie Barany.

(1) "Many of you have never seen a cervix before"; (2) "I think mine is beautiful"; (3) "I want to show you that there are no teeth in there"; and (4) "There was a time that women couldn't wear skirts above their ankles, then they wore miniskirts. This is the next step." She then reveals a "standard, gynecological, metal speculum" which she inserts, feigning surprise over the "tightness of her pussy." She invites the audience to line up in front of the raised stage so that each one may see her cervix. Her male assistant holds a flashlight which he hands to each approaching viewer. Those interested bend down and shine the flashlight onto the exposed cervix while Sprinkle holds a microphone near their mouth, soliciting and broadcasting reactions to this spectacle (see Figures 26 and 27). She asks them to describe what they see so that those who don't have a chance can at least hear about it. The line eventually ends, Sprinkle takes out the speculum, signaling the PCA's completion, and the show's intermission begins.

In "Post Post Porn Modernist" the PCA is sandwiched between a series of vignettes that explore sex, specifically the politics, constructions, pains, and pleasures of being a woman and a porn star. The first is titled "Ellen/Annie," in which Sprinkle discusses her past as Ellen Steinberg and how she became Annie Sprinkle, followed by "Some Basic Background Information," a performative illustration of the construction of a porn star; Sprinkle discusses her transformation as she makes adjustments to her voice and adds a wig, high heels, and so on. She carries this porn persona into "Annie's Toy Chest," in which she shares her favorite sex toys. Then the audience is invited "On the Set with Annie Sprinkle" and is encouraged to help Sprinkle play with her favorite sex toy, the camera, by using their own cameras (which a few hard-core fans have brought) to photograph her as she positions herself in classic porn poses, including the ever-popular "split beaver." Sprinkle transforms out of porn persona and into analytical mode to share her "Pornstistics," accompanied by slides such as "Amount of Dick Sucked," which pictures a large penis graphed alongside the Empire State Building. In "100 Blow Jobs" Sprinkle sucks a variety of dildos affixed to a board until she gags; meanwhile, a sound recording booms degrading phrases such as "Suck it, you bitch" or "Yeah, I bought you dinner—you should suck my cock!" Sprinkle recovers from this while preparing for the "Bosom Ballet," donning a bright red tutu and baring her breasts. To a classic ballet melody she manipulates them as though they are the dancers and she the puppeteer. The PCA is next. Following that is "Tits on Your Head"; for $5 an audience member can take home his or her very own Polaroid with Sprinkle's tits on his or her head. After intermission, the show continues with a question-and-answer session and a slide catalogue of a variety of Sprinkle's sexual partners, many of whom have died of AIDS. The performance climaxes with Sprinkle's transformation into Anya, a sacred prostitute goddess, whose blissful vibrator-induced orgasms finish the show.

Much can be (and has been) said about Sprinkle's one-woman show: critically, historically, and theoretically. I have offered a brief description of the whole performance in an attempt to contextualize the focal point of this chapter—the "Public Cervix Announcement." In fact, "Post Post Porn Modernist" is only the PCA's most recent residence. When it was first performed at "Smutfest" in New York in the early 1980s, it was a piece unto itself. Even within "Post Post Porn Modernist" the PCA stands apart from the rest of the show due to its employment of medical technology, its staging, and its traditionally underpornographed spectacle (a cervix).

Sprinkle's cervical act raises a number of interesting questions: How do codes of medicine, art, and pornography function within the PCA? What aspects of actual gynecological practice does the PCA highlight, critique, or reinscribe? Likewise, how may the PCA function as pornography? as alternative feminist health practice? How does a theatrical mode of representation alter cervical display, and vice versa? Taking Sprinkle's four performed reasons for her act of cervical display as organizational headings for a historical, critical, and theoretical investigation of the "Public Cervix Announcement," I will draw on two interviews conducted with Sprinkle in an attempt to address these questions.[1] These cited interviews are not meant to offer any "truer" glimpse of the PCA, nor to privilege

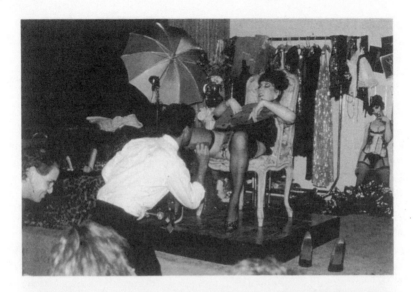

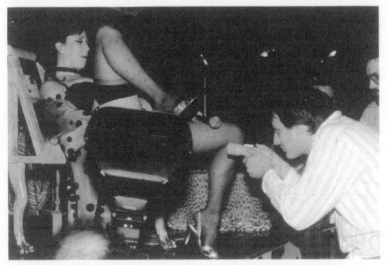

Figure 26. On the set with Sprinkle during the "Public Cervix Announcement."
Photo by Leslie Barany.
Figure 27. Man viewing Sprinkle's cervix with a flashlight while Sprinkle holds a
microphone during the "Public Cervix Announcement." Photo by Leslie Barany.

Sprinkle's stated intentions for the PCA over other critical readings. Nor would the elimination of Sprinkle's discussion of the PCA lead to a more critical investigation of her performance. Rather interviews with Sprinkle are used as yet another layer of discourse in this consideration of the PCA.

"Many of You Have Never Seen a Cervix Before"

With this statement, the politics of *seeing* a cervix are immediately called into question. Why have many of you never seen a cervix before? Medical practitioners have traditionally been a privileged audience to cervixes, having access to the necessary technology for inspection: the speculum. Most women have not seen their own cervix, let alone handled a speculum within a classic exam scenario. And yet in the PCA a speculum appears in the hands of a performance artist–porn star. Sprinkle does not recall exactly how it got there: "I remember somehow I ended up with a speculum. In my days of kinky sex, sex clubs, and wild sex parties I think I might have bought it at a sex toy shop. Either that or my gynecologist gave me one. I can't remember which." The speculum as sex toy. Confusing her gynecologist's office with a sex toy shop exemplifies the "seduction of boundaries" that Chris Straayer attributes to Sprinkle.[2] Sprinkle calls attention to the possible uses for the speculum, as gynecologist's tool and as sex toy. Like many other sex toys, it penetrates, but does so in order to promote what Sprinkle calls an "eye fuck." ("I loved the sensation of eyes looking inside.") In this sense, the speculum participates in an ocular economy similar to Sprinkle's other favorite sex gadget, the camera (see Figure 28). The camera and the speculum, whether used for pornographic, artistic, or medical purposes (or any combination of the three), are used in order to display sex, in order to visualize the "materiality" of female sex. This visualization may locate the point at which the tenuous division between such distinct modes of display collapse.

Although the seed for the PCA was planted in the privacy of Sprinkle's bedroom in the form of a sex game with her lover, it has grown into a different kind of play: "The piece for me now is like little kids playing doctor . . . The first time I did the Public Cervix Announcement was when I was scheduled to perform at the Harmony Burlesque Theater. I had nothing planned. I saw the speculum, grabbed it and the performance hasn't really changed much since then. It's not about sex, it's about 'Pull down your panties, let's look inside.'" The notion of "playing doctor" suggests an innocent complicity in visualizing secret body parts. However, playing doctor is also a power play. Playing doctor quenches a simultaneously naive and "dirty" curiosity, while invoking and appropriating the codes of medical viewing and knowledge.

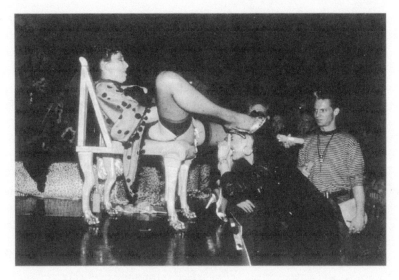

Figure 28. Woman photographing Sprinkle's cervix during the "Public Cervix Announcement." Photo by Leslie Barany.

Sprinkle's initial public rendering of the PCA took the classic gynecological scenario of male practitioner and female patient into account. Her friend Diane Tore, cross-dressing as a man with a drawn mustache, inserted the speculum while Sprinkle performed the role as patient. But a woman obviously *costumed* as a man inserting a speculum into another woman operates differently than an actual man inserting a speculum. As Butler notes, "What drag exposes, however, is the 'normal' constitution of gender presentation in which the gender performed is in many ways constituted by a set of disavowed attachments or identifications that constitute a different domain of the 'unperformable.'"[3] The normal constitution of gender presentation in gynecology is that of male practitioner and female spectacle. A cross-dressing female practitioner highlights this traditional gendered relationship. Such gender play at once calls attention to the implied and performed gender and power position of (s)he who penetrates with the speculum, creating the space for the "eye fuck."

The mystique of the speculum and the fear and anxiety surrounding its use help maintain this powered relationship between the practitioner-penetrator and patient-penetrated. Sprinkle's performance is linked technologically to the very tool that J. Marion Sims, the Father of Gynecology, helped develop. Whereas Sims initially used the speculum in order to perform surgeries on slave women, Sprinkle uses the very same tool to comment on the display of female bodies in medicine, art, and pornography. The speculum's history of pain has continued into its present-day reputation. For many women, the speculum is a tool that signifies fear and discomfort. Sprinkle says that the part of the PCA that gets the "worst reaction" is when she reveals the speculum for the first time: "I take the speculum out and I say, 'I'm going to use this standard gynecological speculum' and all these women go [she closes her eyes, grits her teeth] like they're really uncomfortable just seeing a speculum. That's the hardest part. They go 'Owwww,' like they're really uncomfortable." The speculum serves as a metonym for the pain and discomfort that many women associate with a gynecological exam. In the PCA's nascent days, Sprinkle herself was subject to similar fears: "The first couple of times I did it I felt like there was an air of danger, but now I don't have that sense at all. Somehow I thought I might be vulnerable to some kind of violence or something. I had a fear of the speculum itself, that someone might grab it out or push it in . . . Or a fear of people's reactions." It was a male director, Emilia Cubeiro, who suggested to the intravaginal performance pioneer that she insert the speculum herself during the performance. At first Sprinkle resisted. "I told him I couldn't, it was too hard . . . but now it's the most comfortable, natural thing in the world, like showing the bottom of my foot." The transition from cross-dressing technician to self-insertion has clearly changed the meaning of the PCA. This progression is comparable to the feminist self-help movement's amendment to the classic exam scenario. Whereas traditionally a professional clinician inserts the speculum, in a self-help exam a woman learns how to insert her own speculum in an attempt to regain some degree of control over this very vulnerable experience. For the women in Sprinkle's audience who overwhelmingly identify the speculum with bodily pain, is this changeover from practitioner-insertion to self-insertion simply synonymous with a transition from sadistic to masochistic performance?

Women in Sprinkle's audience, for whom the first view of the clanky speculum revives bodily memories of anxiety-ridden (or even painful) past examinations, potentially have a different idea about the speculum and its uses by the end of the PCA. By making the often terrifying and private experience of a speculum exam a public spectacle, Sprinkle may seriously alter conceptions of the exam by demystifying medical machinery and female bodies, aims of the feminist self-help movement as well. The mystery and power associated with wielding a speculum help perpetuate women patients' anxieties. Following Sprinkle's performance of self-insertion and extended cervical display, the speculum, a benign instrument, may thus no longer serve as terrifying trope. Instead the PCA could point to the fact that it is not the speculum that is inherently horrifying, but rather other aspects of the exam that cause fear and even harm. While it is possible that women feel pain during a speculum exam, it need not be a painful experience if proper emotional support and physical treatment accompany it. It is not the nature of the tool itself, not the gynecological technology, but rather its (mis)use that generally causes pain.

On the other hand, perhaps Sprinkle's performance does not serve to extricate the pain from the tool. Maybe the speculum not only maintains its torturous connotations, but is also given the added connotation of pleasure—pleasurable both for the performer as Sprinkle moans while inserting it and pleasurable for the sadistically oriented viewer who reads Sprinkle's moans as both pleasure and pain. Sprinkle's performance may thus feed institutional and popular fantasies of the oversexed gynecology patient who gets sexual gratification from the exam. Does Sprinkle's PCA simply provide audience members with sadistic fantasy ingredients? What are the politics of sexualizing this tool that so many women find distasteful, but to which so many women are subject at least once a year?

Seeing a cervix in the context of Sprinkle's PCA requires two acts: inserting the speculum and looking into the vagina. It shares these acts with the classic medical speculum exam. In addition, the medical exam usually includes a collection of samples or smears, and it also presupposes that the spectator-audience-clinician has a specific knowledge base. The PCA, on the other hand, presupposes that the spectator–audience member has no specific knowledge base but rather a novice curiosity. The PCA is not a diagnostic exam during which the cervical viewer searches for pathology. Rather it is more like a self-help exam during which pathology may be noticed, but where emphasis is placed on viewing normal, healthy anatomy. Even if an audience member were a medical clinician with a working knowledge of gynecology, it is unlikely that a traditional exam scenario could evolve during the PCA. Its staging positions Sprinkle as controlling the performance. Audience members are relegated to the position of ineffectual onlookers who do what they are told, as opposed to the traditional role of clinicians who serve as directors, exercising control over the exam.

The staging of the PCA is not completely unlike the staging of a traditional gynecological exam. Theatrically, the PCA exists on two simultaneous and interactive levels. There is the larger mise-en-scène, bounded by the space of the stage, in which Sprinkle moves and speaks, dresses and undresses. Then there is a mini mise-en-scène that is formed with the propping open of her vagina and the display of her cervix. Vaginal walls and cervix serve as a little makeshift medical diorama or peep show, bracketed by the speculum. Even the manner in which the tiny spectacle is viewed—one person at a time, peering into opened space—brings to mind a little stage. Some women complain that when they are examined the spectator-clinician ignores the larger for the mini mise-en-scène; the clinician focuses so intensely upon the little internal stage that the larger performance (including the woman's thoughts and feelings about the situation) are disregarded. Various clinical props—footrests, drape sheet, medical lamp, table position, to name a few—foster the clinician's ability to dismiss the larger mise-en-scène in order to focus on the mini mise-en-scène.

However, these clinical props are noticeably absent from the PCA. Sprinkle does not sport a medical gown and drape sheet that would segment her body for proper clinical presentation. Rather she wears sexy porn star gear that confuses the boundaries of clinical conduct. Likewise, her upright bodily position allows her to look back at her spectators, which she does as she actively engages her audience through words, eye contact, and attitude. In addition, within the PCA the spectators viewing Sprinkle's cervix are continually reminded of the larger mise-en-scène via the methods Sprinkle uses in her performance. If spectators venture forth to view Sprinkle's cervix, they are in fact incorporated into the performance. They are handed a flashlight, since no lamp or spotlight is in place, and they must get fairly close to Sprinkle and the speculum in order to see her cervix. Sprinkle's strategic use of the microphone, enlisting viewers to comment on and describe her cervix, encourages spectators to shift focus continually between the larger and the mini mise-en-scène, making it difficult for them to focus constant and undivided attention on her internal anatomy. Thus in the PCA there are multiple performances occurring simultaneously and juggled masterfully. Sprinkle negotiates the audience's attention; they are made to focus both on Sprinkle's internal parts and on her semiscripted thoughts and revelations. In addition, the audience's spoken interpretations and comments are incorporated into the performance. Unlike in most clinical exams, Sprinkle encourages verbal exchange rather than distanced spectatorship. And contrary to the conventional clinical model, Sprinkle, the object of the gaze, initiates such conversational exchange. Thus, given the workings of this performance, it is doubtful that the PCA simply promotes ideas about the speculum as sadistic pleasure tool since Sprinkle remains comfortable and relaxed with the speculum in place and converses freely with her audience. She is not concerned with staging speculum-derived pain, but instead inserts an insistent rhetoric into the PCA that promotes her personal agenda for cervical display, one which, among other things, professes the beauty of the cervix and the potential pleasures of viewing it.

"I Think Mine Is Beautiful"

This statement is directly linked to the mission of the women's self-help health movement that began in the late 1960s and early '70s. In response to cultural institutions, like commercial advertising, which simultaneously oversexualize the female body and maintain taboos on menstruation and vaginal "odor," and medicine, which persistently pathologizes women's bodies, this movement works toward self-empowerment for women by advocating knowledge about one's own body. Women are encouraged to view their bodies as beautiful rather than flawed or ugly. Cervical self-exam using a speculum, mirror, and flashlight is suggested by self-helpers as a way to demystify the unknown "down there."

Sprinkle sells plastic speculums at her show, rallying women to "show all [their] friends. It's great at parties!" She parodically refers to speculums as though they were Tupperware, lifting some of the seriousness from self-help rhetoric. But Sprinkle shares the philosophical mission of taking the cervix public with self-helpers who themselves have deprivatized the act of cervical viewing by establishing self-help groups where women look at each other's cervixes. Even more public than the self-help group, self-helpers have, like Sprinkle, taken cervical display on the road. The film *Taking Our Bodies Back: The Women's Health Movement* (1974) documents an early performance of cervical display. In the film, a health educator, Jennifer Burgess, speaks to an auditorium filled with young white women, educating them about cervical self-exam. She then lies on a table, inserts the speculum, and invites the women to come up on stage to view her cervix.

I described this ancestral incarnation of the PCA to Sprinkle. She responded, "That's great to hear. I knew I didn't invent it . . . Well, as far as performance art goes I've never heard of anybody doing it." Sprinkle's statement may point to an important difference between her PCA and this other version from the early 1970s. Sprinkle is a performance artist with a paying audience of men and women who have come to see a performance. When she states that her cervix is beautiful, Sprinkle may be referring to it as an art object, aestheticizing that part of her body for public consumption. Sprinkle could also be playing on notions of beauty as manifested in beauty pageants. In this postmodern beauty contest, the swimsuit and talent competitions would be followed by the cervical show-down. In this sense, Sprinkle could be commenting on the aestheticization of individual female body parts. If there is such focus on female breasts, faces and buttocks, what about the cervix?

Certainly Sprinkle's PCA can, at the same time, be about the kind of beauty promoted by the women's health movement. Both she and self-helpers advocate a nonpathology-focused, pro-genital-based consideration of women's bodies. Interestingly, Sprinkle had no direct involvement with the kind of self-help group pictured in the film. She first heard about such groups in the 1970s, but had had a different kind of all-female health empowerment experience: "Being a hooker and hanging out in whorehouses. You share all your stories of your dis-

eases and your warts. You get a real good education about bodies and gynecological things." However, such an open discussion of disease and pathology in the
context of sexual activity is exactly what is missing from the self-help feminist
text *New View of a Woman's Body* discussed in the previous chapter. Sprinkle's
mission is similar to that of the authors of *NVWB*, who, in redefining the clitoris, encouraging cervical self-exam, and stressing variation in healthy anatomy,
contradict the standard medical model. However, whereas *NVWB* barely addresses pathology, Sprinkle turns to pathology elsewhere in her performance by
showing slides of various diseased and disabled lovers (with AIDS, missing
limbs, neurological disorders, etc.). Sprinkle engages in an eroticization of disease and disability, proclaiming that she has found pleasure with these sexual
partners despite or even due to their pathologies. She transgresses prevalent cultural ideas that associate health with beauty and illness with ugliness.[4] Whereas
NVWB entirely associates wellness with beauty and sexiness, Sprinkle performatively associates wellness *and* illness with beauty and sexiness. But Sprinkle
does adhere to certain aesthetic protocols regarding proper bodily presentation.
For instance, the cervix must be cleansed before the PCA.

It was from being a prostitute that Sprinkle began douching for public consumption: "Most people are grossed out by the smell of pussy. When you're a
prostitute a lot of people want you clean and shiny. I used to douche all the time
as a prostitute. . . . You're a commodity, you have to be what they want you to
be." Sprinkle's douching on stage before inserting the speculum is in itself an in-
triguing spectacle.[5] It also prepares the vaginal space and cervix for public viewing, making it "clean and shiny" for the consumer–audience member.

Given Sprinkle's performative choices, the cervix is not necessarily "beautiful" as is, but needs to be "costumed" or prepared for display, stripped of healthy,
normal secretions in order to aestheticize it properly. This does not follow the
women's health movement's credo of discouraging women from douching for
nonmedicinal purposes, educating them instead about the important cleansing
qualities of normal discharge while fighting against the douche industry's fabri-
cated notions of feminine hygiene. Perhaps making a cervix palatable is a justi-
fiable sacrifice if it encourages people not to fear female anatomy. And a "clean
and shiny" cervix may not only be an issue of aesthetics, but of practical performativity. A cervix is simply not as easy to identify and view if it is partially obscured by normal discharge.

Making the cervix clearly visible is part of Sprinkle's pedagogical mission. She
takes on the role of an educator in the PCA, as well as in much of her film, video,
and performance work. Her video, *Sluts and Goddesses* (cocreated with Maria
Beatty, 1992), is a "how-to" piece for female sexual and spiritual pleasure that in-

cludes a short clip of a woman with speculum in place, engaging in cervical self-exam. Whereas *Deep Inside Annie Sprinkle* (1981) is closer to straight-up porn on the hard-core continuum, it also has a pedagogical twist. Sprinkle directly addresses the home viewer in the second person, discussing how she gets off and how "you" might too. Sprinkle's work in general highlights the educational functions of a porn star, prostitute, and performance artist.

If we consider a porn star and performance artist as a health and sex educator, might we consider a health educator a porn star and performance artist? Jennifer Burgess in the film *Taking Our Bodies Back* is certainly on stage, displaying her body. But Burgess does not "play doctor" in the same way as Sprinkle. The pleasures of looking are disavowed within Burgess's cervical display, and instead the empowering reward of knowledge is emphasized. In Sprinkle's PCA, on the contrary, the pleasure of looking is central to her discourse. But how separable are knowledge and pleasure with regard to looking at bodies? Can they be policed in such a way that the quality of the performance, be it executed by a health educator or a porn star, determines the outcome of knowledge *or* pleasure?

Do the economics of the situation help determine the outcome? In the context of the PCA, Sprinkle addresses a paying audience. In "Pornstistics," she is up front about the economic benefits of sex work, and "Post Post Porn Modernist" has a hefty ticket price. It is unclear whether Burgess receives payment. However, the focus of Burgess's performance is not on her own profit, but on the education of a curious audience. In this sense Sprinkle may be more closely aligned with the gynecology teaching associate, who receives payment for using her own body as teaching tool. But the fact that Sprinkle, like the GTA, receives payment for cervical display does not necessarily determine the audience's understanding of the performance as pleasurable or educational.

Does the gender makeup of the audience determine the outcome? Whereas Sprinkle's early work has largely educated a heterosexual male public, Burgess's instance of cervical display is intended for an all-female audience where the possibilities of pleasure and desire are supposedly disavowed in favor of a desexualized medical discourse. Of course, the potential for desire and pleasure in looking at female bodies is possible regardless of the audience member's gender. Sprinkle depends on this possibility in "Post Post Porn Modernist" and *Sluts and Goddesses*, which have transgressed the boundaries of mainstream pornography to allow for and, at times, focus on lesbian and bisexual desire. Thus, an all-female paying audience would still provide the space for Sprinkle's mixture of desire, pleasure, aestheticization, and education. Spectators do not completely define the role of the performer. While Sprinkle's and Burgess's actions (placing the speculum in the vagina, inviting audience members to view the cervix) are almost identical, a delicate mix of tone, language, circumstance, personal history, economics, setting, costume, and advertisement distinguish the very similar acts performed by a performance artist–porn star and a health educator. Nevertheless, the overlap is significant and telling. Both encourage cervical display and cervical self-exam, viewing them as empowering experiences.

According to Sprinkle, her presentation of the cervix as beautiful elicits positive responses from her audiences: "They're lovely, they all smile. It's a great position to be in. Nobody ever goes 'uck' or thinks it's ugly. I get a lot of 'oh that's beautiful' and a lot of thank yous." Undoubtedly, there are those audience members who pass on a cervical view, and some who do view but do not find the cervix beautiful. Sprinkle believes that the knowledge that the PCA will be performed at all probably prevents some from attending "Post Post Porn Modernist." Thus, even though Sprinkle emphasizes the beauty of a cervix, the opposite tension is also present; her performance partially depends upon a deep cultural horror of what is inside, a terror of female genitals and the space behind them. Although Sprinkle assures us that "mine is beautiful," she also hints at the lurking dangers of the vagina.

"I Want to Show You That There Are No Teeth in There"

With this comment Sprinkle refers to widespread fears about vaginas, particularly the mythological "vagina dentata." Numerous cultures have some version of the notion that there are teeth in the vagina, representing a fear of penile insertion, birth, or rebirth. Barbara Creed observes that Freud failed to discuss the vagina dentata in relation to castration anxiety: "To argue that the Medusa's severed head symbolizes the terrifying *castrated* female genitals, and that the snakes represent her fetishized and comforting imaginary phallus, is an act of wish fulfillment *par excellence*. Freud's interpretation masks the active, terrifying aspects of the female genitals—the fact that they might castrate. The Medusa's entire visage is alive with images of toothed vaginas, poised and waiting to strike. No wonder her male victims were rooted to the spot with fear."[6] In Creed's terms, the sight of the woman with her vulva (read: missing penis) is not only a continual reminder to the boy or man that his could be taken from him. The vulva simultaneously represents a monstrous, devouring place that threatens those penises that dare to enter. Not only is the lacking, envious woman the reminder of castration; she is also the emasculating cause.

Sprinkle assures her audience that this is not the case, at least so far as *her* vagina is concerned. The PCA not only offers the new experience of viewing a beautiful cervix, but sets out to disprove damaging labia libel. But by invoking the possibility of vaginal teeth, is Sprinkle legitimating the very possibility? The proof, then, is in the display. In this case, vaginal viewing is perhaps not the horrifying foundation of castration anxiety, but rather comforting evidence to the contrary. Does Sprinkle's "teeth" statement then humorously serve to lessen viewer anxiety? Or might she be playing on the sexy horror of the possibility? (Well, there *could* be teeth in there.)

Sprinkle's audience members are called upon to see for themselves. And, as promised, there are no teeth to be seen. But the first handful of audiences that viewed the PCA within the "Post Post Porn Modernist" context must not have been expecting anything other than the reassurance that no teeth were there, because no cervix was visible either. Sprinkle was new at inserting the speculum and did not realize that it could be comfortably in place with the cervix trapped behind a speculum bill, out of view: "Hundreds of people thought they were seeing my cervix and no one ever said anything. Chances are that half the time you couldn't see it at all." The expectation for an empty space was met, entire audiences gazing without comment "deep inside Annie Sprinkle" into a black hole. Were these audience members satisfied simply by the evidence that "there are no teeth in there"? The expectation of an empty hole was quietly confirmed by Sprinkle's PCA.

The first night I saw the PCA, Sprinkle's "clean and shiny" cervix was in plain view. Most audience members did step up to Sprinkle's cervical altar, gazing into the speculum with flashlight in hand, uttering comments like "Wow," "Beautiful," or "Thank you." Two white male audience members responded differently, their reactions broadcast via Sprinkle's microphone. Commenting on Sprinkle's cervix, one said, "It looks like the head of the penis." Sprinkle agreed, "Yeah, it kind of does." Another further down the line offered, "I can see myself in it." Sprinkle giggled, "That's because it's so clean and shiny."

These two respondents are exemplary caricatures of Luce Irigaray's critique of male spectatorship in *Speculum of the Other Woman*. Irigaray explores how woman has been made simultaneously "other," negative, and mirror-image of man, leaving her outside of representation and discourse. For Irigaray, the word "speculum" takes on a multiplicity of meanings, including the instrument used by gynecologists and Sprinkle, as well as that of a mirror. The very shape of the concave, reflecting speculum morphologically imitates the object it mirrors, the cavernous vagina: "*But this cave is already, and ipso facto, a speculum. An inner space of reflection. Polished, and polishing, fake offspring. Opening, enlarging, contriving the scene of representation, the world as representation. All is organized into cavities, spheres, sockets, chambers, enclosures, simply because the speculum is put in the way.*"[7] Representation and truth are structured by the visual. Spectatorship is gendered with male spectators subject to what Toril Moi calls a "specular logic of the same."[8] They use a space, in this case the cavity of the female vagina, for self-reflection and self-contemplation.

One might insist that the two male respondents commenting on Sprinkle's cervix were simply offering innocent descriptions. While this could be true, these men do illustrate Irigaray's ideas, serving almost as comic or hyperbolic incarnations of those masters who are viewing with the "blind spot of an old dream of symmetry,"[9] finding self-reflection ("I can see myself in it") while engaging in self-contemplation ("It looks like the head of a penis"). Of course, they are relating their first vaginal view to what is familiar to them. But one might justly ask how many women upon seeing a penis would say, "Oh that looks just like a cervix."

Here I am at risk of oversimplifying Irigaray's beautiful and complex arguments. It is interesting, however, that at many times throughout her piece she directly refers to vulvas and vaginas. Reflecting on Freud's treatises on femininity, Irigaray muses, "Now the little girl, the woman, supposedly has *nothing* you can see. She exposes, exhibits the possibility of a *nothing to see*."[10] Though "there are no teeth in there," Sprinkle offers us the view past the vulva (a common pornographic and classic art trope that Freudians and Lacanians construct as "lacking" or *nothing*) to yet another place where there is indeed something to be seen, an idea suggested by Irigaray's tone. The very act of cervical display and the focusing of the viewer's attention onto the cervix challenges the same notions that Irigaray contests with her biting prose.

In presenting her cervix for display, does Sprinkle still remain outside of discourse and representation, letting "ones," particularly white male audience members, with access to phallocratic discourse "speak" while "others are silent"?[11] Irigaray herself has been criticized for her notion that women are outside discourse. How then is she writing a book?[12] Or is she not a woman, but a woman masquerading as a man by engaging in philosophical-speak? Sprinkle too is offering a representation for public viewing. Instead of writing she uses her body as representation, constructing discourse through her cervical display. Is she engaging in phallocratic discourse by *accepting* the respondents' descriptions? (Man 1: It looks like the head of a penis. Sprinkle: Yeah, it kind of does; Man 2: I can see myself in it. Sprinkle: That's because it's so clean and shiny.) Or, by agreeing with the men, by comforting them into speaking, does she allow them to reveal their own discursive limitations? It is possible that these two male respondents were playfully engaging Sprinkle by improvising their own parodic responses to the PCA. They even could have been self-aware of the patriarchal inflections of their cervical interpretations. Perhaps they were refusing to be positioned as worshippers at Sprinkle's cervix, acquiescing with generic responses of admiration, and instead formed new responses as a form of resistance. If nothing else, these men were speaking up and acknowledging the fact that there is indeed a cervix to be discussed.

Not only does Sprinkle show that "there are no teeth in there," but she also dispels the foundational myth that there is *nothing* to be seen. Rather she provides evidence for those that venture forth to gaze into the speculum that there *is* a cervix in there. Perhaps she sidesteps the incessant discourse of "have" and "have not," of "presence" and "lack," as does Mister Rogers with his pioneering lyrics:

> Boys are fancy on the outside
> Girls are fancy on the inside
> Everybody's fancy
> Everybody's fine.
> Your body's fancy
> And so is mine.

However, not every spectator is open to viewing Sprinkle's fancy insides. Whether out of fear or distaste, Sprinkle says that "a lot of people, they just pass by real quick and I know they're not seeing my cervix and I always have to say 'No you didn't see it, you just saw the vaginal walls, and the vaginal walls are kind of dull. Make sure you see the cervix.'" Though the cervix is undoubtedly billed as the star of the PCA, it does not always get the recognition Sprinkle expects. "Sometimes people are a little disappointed. There's sometimes a 'so what' reaction. They're expecting . . . I don't know *what* they're expecting [she laughs]." What is expected? Is the cervix not performative enough?

The very title of the piece "Public Cervix Announcement" points to the idea that Sprinkle is presenting her cervix as though it is an active participant, placing it on its speculum-podium so that it may announce to the world that it exists. An obvious play on "public service announcement," the connection here is that Sprinkle constructs the PCA as an educational service to her audience. The word "announcement" in particular plays into the frequent discussions of speech act theory among gender theorists, particularly those concerned with performance, such as Judith Butler and Eve Kosofsky Sedgwick.[13] The "announcement" does not exclusively refer to the words emanating from Sprinkle's mouth. Rather the act of inserting the speculum and displaying her cervix may be viewed as a constitutive utterance, one that emanates from a different set of lips. Sprinkle's "announcement" is a performative action that may help constitute the materiality of sex and gender in new and interesting ways.

The "Public Cervix Announcement" can be considered part of a genre of Sprinkle's work that is typified by the creation of a body-based mini mise-en-scène to house the theatrical animation of specific body parts. The "Bosom Ballet" described at the beginning of this chapter operates in a similar manner. The audience is expected to focus on Sprinkle's breasts as she maneuvers them through a short duet. Sprinkle is adept at figuring out different ways of using her body as an active performance tool. She also creates bodily spectacle by using her muscles and fluids: "I've been doing this little performance. The first time, I wanted to shoot ping pong balls out of my pussy. I showed one of my old golden shower movies. It was like a film festival and then I did a shoulder stand and I spread my legs open and I was going to become a sprinkling sparkling fountain. I drank all this water and I had an assistant (who happened to be a midwife) put sparklers in my boots and she'd plug a ping pong ball into my pussy and it would just roll down. It wouldn't shoot out, but it didn't matter. I could squirt cause I could pee and hit the ceiling in a shoulder stand position if I drink tons of water. It's just like this huge fountain. Everyone loved it because people are amazed that you can pee upside down." Sprinkle repeated this performance at the Gay and Lesbian March on Washington '93, where she became the "DuPont Circle Fountain," adding birds and candles to the routine. Sprinkle's performances often have an air of bodily stunt work.[14] Her video performance of female ejaculation in *Sluts and Goddesses* shows another commitment to portraying the breadth of *activity* available to the female body. Once again, the "nothing to see" is turned into something to see *and* do (e.g., shooting urine or ejaculate).[15] This could be why some audience members are disappointed at their eventual view of Sprinkle's cervix: it really doesn't *do* much of anything. Sprinkle doesn't make it dance or wave. The activity of the cervix doesn't compare to the kinds of activity Sprinkle's performances commonly adopt. The pleasure of peeing a strong stream or of ejaculating, primarily male pleasures, are appropriated by Sprinkle frequently in her performances. Activity and pleasure go hand in hand. Activity is evidence of pleasure.

This is yet another part of Sprinkle's performative proposal for a new "materiality" of sex for women, one that suggests alternatives to the traditional binaries that ally passivity with femininity and activity with masculinity. Although Sprinkle's cervix does not mimic the kind of active performance discussed, the PCA challenges narrow and normative assumptions regarding female sexuality and beauty. It calls into question the way the codes of medicine, art, and pornography situate the female body, more specifically the cervix. By taking an active role in promoting the display of her cervix as an educational experience for her audience, Sprinkle pushes ideas of proper female performance, medical or otherwise. In doing so, she contradicts the primary ways that the materiality of sex has been forcibly produced in the context of medical cervical display: model female spectacle as passive and pathological.

*"There Was a Time When Women Couldn't
Wear Skirts above Their Ankles; Then They
Wore Mini-Skirts. This Is the Next Step."*

Representations, fears, and myths surrounding vulvas and vaginas are in continual flux and transformation on cultural and historical levels. Sprinkle discusses some of these changes in terms of advertising: "I've noticed big changes in bathing suit ads. Now they're letting the pussy crack show. Before, women always had their legs one in front of the other, they never showed it. Just recently they're beginning to let it show. It's a small step but it's something." Sprinkle actively supports what might be termed "pussy liberation." According to her, such revolutionary activity seeks the visibility of both female genitals and feminist activism. On my second visit with Sprinkle, she presented me with a Women's Health Action Movement button which reads "Support Vaginal Pride." Pussy liberation is simultaneously an earnest and excessive enterprise. Likewise, Sprinkle's performance and video works often cross the boundaries of pornography, extending into a new territory—a medico-porn-kitsch place where excess presides. Sprinkle performatively turns her body inside out, showing her audience that there are no teeth in there, but there is a cervix. A cervix may be for some a "vision of excess," like Bataille's big toe or, more appropriately, the mouth (a place that is both inside and outside and has teeth of its own).[16] The very act of cervical display is in itself excessive. Thus Sprinkle is a performative realization of what Mary Russo refers to as a "female grotesque," presenting an "open, protruding," abject, and oozing body in a spectacular display.[17]

Sprinkle herself is aware of this "grotesque" potential: "In some ways the Public Cervix Announcement is a 'fuck you' to the guys who came to see pussy. 'You want to see pussy, I'll show you pussy.' I want to gross them out. It's a slap in the face." Sprinkle is undressing pornography, seeking out points of excess that might unbalance the assumed porn equation of active pleasure-seeker and passive model-spectacle in an attempt to make certain members in her audience uncomfortable. In her work, pornographic and medical acts are often placed side by side or even collapsed. Sprinkle draws on these two visual economies that privilege both excess and sensational anomalies. For instance, Sprinkle's video *Linda, Les, and Annie: The First Female-to-Male Transsexual Love Story* (created with Al Jaccoma and Johnny Armstrong, 1990) is simultaneously a sex story, medical story, and love story. The blurb on the video box's cover reads like a cross between a Ripley's Believe It or Not tabloid, a carny's pitch, and a made-for-TV medical serial: "A fun, unique, sexy, and informative video docu-drama about Les Nichols, a woman who became a man (and is now actually a surgically made hermaphrodite). It includes an intimate view of the night he and Annie Sprinkle tried out his new, surgically constructed penis for the first time. His dual-genitalia and all of their functions are shown in graphic detail. Revealing interviews and explicit medical photographs have made this film sought after by sex therapists, film buffs, porn fans and connoisseurs of the unusual alike. See it to believe it."

Sprinkle is familiar with the traditional medical establishment and the need to construct important visual spectacle as "unbelievable." In fact, although medical publishers turned down Sprinkle's photograph discussed in the previous chapter, she has sold numerous photographs to medical textbooks. The ones the publishers bought were actually of Les Nichols's genitals and surgery. But they were interested in an assortment of bodily anomalies, "enlarged clitorises, hermaphrodites, unusual breast sizes, scars." Sprinkle is well aware of the number of ways in which the sex world and the medical industry intermingle: "I have friends in the porn industry that model for Kotex or Tampax. They go in there and the guys that design fit them with their stuff. My friends say the guys totally get off on it. Oh, and they videotape it!" Thus, sex workers serve as both models and frontline image producers for the medical and sanitary hygiene industries. Similarly, Sprinkle, a famous sex worker, porn star, and performance artist, not only sells her photos to medical publishers but also adopts the very sensational and excessive act of cervical exam into her staged performance, exemplifying the porous boundaries between medicine, pornography, and art.

Sprinkle's last reason for performing the PCA rhetorically points to the different levels at which this medical act operates within a performance art scenario. By creating the bottom-up order of skirts below ankles, miniskirts, then cervical display, Sprinkle creates a mental image of a cone with the cervix at the top. Female internal anatomy becomes the pinnacle of beauty, the newest and bravest of fashion statements. Sprinkle says that she is simply ahead of her time.[18] Considering cervical display as a new fashion accounts for an audience member's possible distaste upon viewing this innovative sight; many people thought miniskirts were ugly when they first saw them, but then they themselves began to wear them. Likewise, Sprinkle encourages women in her audience to join her trendsetting when she suggests they use speculums at parties.

The idea that cervical display is a "next step" has additional connotations. This next step points to the power of bodily display, of revealing a space that is both inside the body and outside representation, a space that is traditionally colonized by the medical establishment and ignored by the porn industry. This "next step" is a political act, maybe even radical and revolutionary.[19] Sprinkle notes that there is a great deal of power in the simplest of actions or displays, "the value of a simple thing like showing your cervix. It can be total liberation."[20] Some feminist critics are uneasy with the way Sprinkle has taken her privates public, believing she is the master of her own objectification.[21] (One might ask if any performance or image, particularly those that privilege the female body, is outside of "objectification.") I believe it is her playful blending of the medical, pornographic, and artistic realms combined with pro-sex, self-help, and pathology-friendly rhetoric that many find unsettling.

Considering the PCA, I have examined the ways cervical display functions aesthetically, medically, and pornographically. In *undressing* pornography, does Sprinkle turn cervical display into a grotesque act? a pleasurable act? an aestheticized act? Does Sprinkle's PCA upset what Butler refers to as the "forcible production" of the "materiality of sex"? Or does it simply reinforce that which is always already forcibly produced? In offering a material representation of the materiality of sex, is Sprinkle hopelessly replicating norms or is she creating something new by chipping away at pornographic and medical representational structures, while simultaneously adopting them in her performance of cervical display? Like most revolutions, the PCA leaves us with a set of questions rather than neatly contained answers.

6 Playing Doctor:
Cronenberg's Surgical Construction
of Mutant Female Bodies

The only reason I played the gynaecologist in *The Fly* was because Geena Davis begged me to. She didn't want a stranger between her legs, and felt more comfortable with me there. And it was a very convenient place to direct the scene from. —David Cronenberg, *Cronenberg on Cronenberg*

(Dr.) Cronenberg

Although he is not a physician, David Cronenberg often situates himself as one when making a film. His science fictive projects are saturated with images of psychologically and physiologically pathologized bodies. In the films *Dead Ringers* (1988), *Rabid* (1976), and *The Brood* (1979), the director relentlessly attends to female bodies and female sexualities and their host of accompanying, and inevitable, illnesses, excesses, and contagions. Cronenberg uses these narrative preoccupations to theorize and rationalize his role as doctor-director: "I am being this clinician, this surgeon, and trying to examine the nature of sexuality. I'm doing it by creating characters I then dissect with my cinematic scalpels."[1] Why does Cronenberg choose to portray himself as a cinematic surgeon? What aspects of the medical apparatus and filmic apparatus and their attendant institutions facilitate this director's appropriation of the title "surgeon"?

Cronenberg is not the first to use medicine as a metaphor for the cinema. In

"The Work of Art in the Age of Mechanical Reproduction," Walter Benjamin compares the art of filmmaking to that of surgery. The magician who heals by "laying on hands" is like the painter, but the surgeon who "penetrates the body of his patient" is closest to the cameraman. The surgeon-cameraman directly manipulates the body, either flesh or celluloid. The surgeon edits the body, repairing or removing organs, rearranging parts, then suturing the body in order to make it whole once again. Similarly, the filmmaker, according to Benjamin, creates a picture of a reality, composed of "multiple fragments which are assembled under a new law."[2] With its hands-on manipulation of the filmic body altering representations of the real, filmmaking is both art and science insofar as it remakes a material world. Benjamin believes that it is film's very connection to art and science that allows it to function as both.

Indeed, Benjamin was not mistaken when he foresaw the use of film in science. And the intricacy of their relationship might be more than he imagined. As Lisa Cartwright states, "The long history of bodily analysis and surveillance in medicine and science is critically tied to the history of the development of the cinema as a popular cultural institution and a technological apparatus."[3] This intimate connection between the cinematic apparatus and science and medicine is not surprising given that modern Western medicine, as Foucault notes, arose with the visualization of pathology. A trend toward more specialized modes of visualization continues. More elaborate visualizing technologies (video, MRI, etc.) continue to be developed and utilized in medicine so that the body becomes even more visibly accessible. With these new technologies Western medicine adheres to the idea so fundamental to its inception, that pathology must be more exactly localized and visualized. And yet such technologies are still contained within the realm of representation. The *material* body, though constituted by such technologies, remains outside of the X ray and the video screen. And yet the viewer of an X ray might be seduced into believing that the image *is* the body, even though it is a representation.[4] Jean Baudrillard's notion of simulation is at play here, just as he assures us it is with regard to medicine; the simulation replaces the signified, the representation is taken for what is real.[5]

Cronenberg's use of the cinema is similar to a clinician's use of visualizing technologies in Western medicine, thus confirming his self-appraisal of cinematic surgeon. With their visualizing apparatuses, both physicians and Cronenberg offer us normally unseen visions of the enemy: the bloody trace of endometriosis or the societal nightmare of an unstoppable, cannibalistic venereal disease (now both available on video for home viewing).[6] One might insist that the doctor and film director are using technology very differently—one creates a reality, one creates a fiction. But what they are doing is actually very similar;

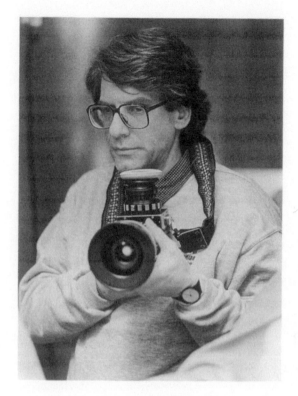

Figure 29. Publicity still
of Cronenberg on the set
of *Dead Ringers.* Photo by
Attila Dory.

both are visualizing or making visual constructions of bodies through which
spectators may access a partial perspective, but never an entire reality. Medicine,
like film, is an interpretive "science" that depends upon visualizing technologies
for its production of truth and knowledge.

   Although Benjamin did discuss the power of film on the unconscious, his notion of the cameraman as surgeon largely rests on the mechanical aspects of film
production. But when Cronenberg discusses his role as cinematic surgeon, he is
not simply discussing the technological manipulations of filmmaking. The metaphor of surgeon also suggests a relationship between Cronenberg and his film
audience. His artful dissections suture his audience into his cinematic science
experiments. The notion of suture in contemporary film theory extends Benjamin's notion of the filmmaker as surgeon to consider the way in which mechanical processes such as shot-reverse-shot editing and the 180-degree rule suture
the spectator into filmic space, stitching the viewer's subjectivity into the film's
narrative. In this notion of suture, production actually becomes invisible to the
viewing subject who no longer sees edit breaks or point-of-view changes. Rather

the viewer perceives a cohesive narrativized space. As Stephen Heath notes, "Meaning, entertainment, vision: film produced as the realization of a coherent and positioned space, and as that realization *in movement*, positioning, cohering, binding in."[7] Cronenberg is a cinematic surgeon not only in his reconfiguring of the filmic body, but also in the sense that he stitches his film audience's subjectivity into narrative space.

There is a third level at which Cronenberg sees himself as surgeon. He considers his films to be science experiments, explorations of the nature of the human mind and body. Cronenberg the surgeon assembles these narratives. He is the director, in the seat of authority, who reconfigures art for science's sake. He confirms Benjamin's notion that film is and represents both art and science by maintaining that his art is scientific art. But this rhetorical costume of cinematic surgeon also affords Cronenberg the ruse of objectivity and scientific distance associated with Western medicine. By labeling himself a filmic physician, Cronenberg legitimates his science fiction creations. Since much power is attached to the medical profession, brandishing the label cinematic surgeon is an act of power, a move intent on "radically" restructuring the filmic, audience, and narrative bodies.[8]

Chris Rodley, the editor of *Cronenberg on Cronenberg*, a book containing long passages from interviews with Cronenberg, also seems intent on validating the director's medical alliances. The foreword of the book is written by Dr. Martyn Steenbeck, a psychologist whose title Dr. is awkwardly prominent. Steenbeck, situated as validating scientific expert, assures the reader that "Cronenberg's practice itself is truly scientific. The films are experiments, conducted in a 'pure' sense, with little or no regard for the consequences."[9] He compares Cronenberg with a "mad scientist," one who sees the world from the disease's perspective. However, Cronenberg's siding with the disease does not reconfigure his connection with scientific values. Cronenberg's "disregard for the consequences" results in filmic science experiments founded on ideological assumptions regarding gender and pathology that also pervade more conventional scientific forms such as biology, psychiatry, and gynecology.

Rodley, in discussing *Dead Ringers* (1988), makes connections between Cronenberg and the two little boys who play the twin gynecologists as youngsters. A photograph showing Cronenberg leaning over the two young boys appears in the book (see Figure 30). All three wear similar glasses and the boys decidedly resemble Cronenberg. The caption under the photo reads, "Return to childhood: Cronenberg directs *Dead Ringers*." The text accompanying the photograph contains Cronenberg's confession: "The kids in *Dead Ringers* are partly modeled after me. I did wear glasses as a kid, I was interested in science and I was preco-

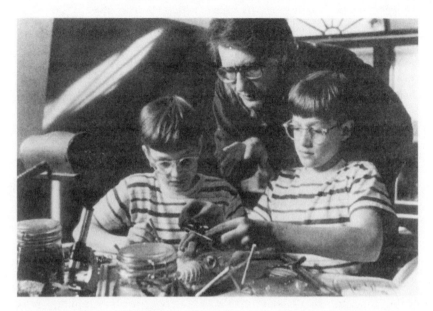

Figure 30. "Return to childhood: Cronenberg directs *Dead Ringers.*" In Chris Rodley, ed. *Cronenberg on Cronenberg.* Boston: Faber and Faber, 1991.

cious."[10] In the opening of *Dead Ringers*, these bespectacled boys discuss the difference between fish reproduction and human reproduction, deciding that there are distinct advantages to contactless underwater spawning. They then ask a little girl classmate of theirs if she will join them in an experiment and have sex with them. She tells them to "fuck off." The next scene shows the twins operating on a toy: a plastic, see-through woman with removable organs they carefully extract with tweezers. The message here is that resistant women (those who tell little boys to "fuck off") must be avoided in lieu of more compliant patient objects (doll-like, passive, plastic models), a preference and pattern that can be located, as we have seen, throughout the history of gynecological practice and pedagogy.

These two scenes serve as an explanation for the twins' desire to become gynecologists; their initial fascination with sex, spawning, and undoubtedly, their own twin origins lead them to become fertility specialists who perform dramatic surgeries on anesthetized women (plastic doll correlates). What starts as an innocent, but already slightly perverse, childhood curiosity in playing doctor is narratively legitimated by the twins' medical and surgical training. This set of introductory scenes also presents some of Cronenberg's initial hypotheses: Men are spectators (they might even wear spectacles). They dissect women, simultaneously intrigued and disgusted by contact with them. The subject of the scientific gaze is gendered male. The object of fascination of that gaze is gendered female. Cronenberg does not call these orthodox structures into question, rather they are the foundations of his scientific platform. He states, "Gynecology is such a beautiful metaphor for the mind/body split. Here it is: the mind of men—or women—trying to understand sexual organs."[11] Cronenberg's gratuitous "or women" cannot mask what is at play here: the idea, so basic to the foundation of Western science, that men examining women is a metaphor for science investigating nature.[12] In this formulation, man is mind and woman is body. But this is only the very first assumption underlying *this* science experiment. *Dead Ringers* reveals much more about the "nature" of men and women, spectator and spectacle, gynecologist and patient.

Film as a medium allows Cronenberg to act out his scientific fantasies, making them into public spectacle. Through his fantasy of "playing doctor"—a compelling longing, recalling the popular kind of child's play sometimes associated with children's first nonsolo sexual activity—Cronenberg creates films focused on mutant female bodies and their performative outbursts. Cronenberg, like Sims and Sprinkle, GTAS and textbook editors, is a performer, a cultural producer who helps configure gynecology.

Mutant Woman as Spectacle

Dead Ringers is the story of Beverly and Elliot Mantle, both skillfully portrayed by Jeremy Irons (See Figure 31). The demise of these successful twin male gynecologists is triggered by actress Claire Niveau's entrance into their closely shared medical and sexual lives. Claire, played by Genevieve Bujold, first appears in the film on the examining table in the lithotomy position—that is, in the familiar pose taken in the pelvic exam, the body draped with heels in footrests, knees open. Elliot, posing as his twin brother Beverly, examines Claire. The twins frequently play this game of interchange in order to experience each other's professional and personal lives. After the examination, Elliot diagnoses Claire as a trifurcate, explaining that she possesses three cervixes that lead to three separate chambers in her uterus. Claire and Elliot then go to lunch together with Claire's agent, Leo. The scene opens as Claire and Leo are discussing problems they are having with producers. Leo offers to tell the producers to "fuck off" because he doesn't want Claire to be humiliated. Claire replies, "I've decided I want to be humiliated." She then immediately turns to Elliot (posing as Beverly) and says, "Tell me about my uterus." Elliot is unphased by Claire's bluntness and answers

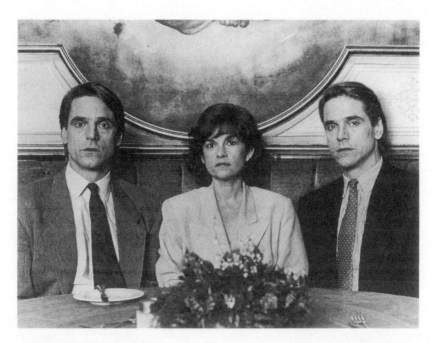

Figure 31. *Dead Ringers* publicity still: Jeremy Irons portraying Beverly Mantle (left) and Elliot Mantle (right) and Genevieve Bujold portraying Claire Niveau. Photo by Attila Dory.

with medical exactitude, but Leo, stunned by Claire's question, chokes on his lunch. When Elliot asks Claire if she has normal periods, Leo begs to be excused. As he leaves, Claire reiterates, "Remember, I need the humiliation as well as the money."

This narrative linking of actresses to humiliation is of particular interest because the actress-character, Claire, is portrayed by Genevieve Bujold, one of the few actresses, according to Cronenberg, who would risk her "reputation" on a role that required she be in "stirrups." That such a role would be considered a career risk suggests a great deal about how women are positioned as gynecology patients. Why would an actress's reputation be at risk because of portraying a gynecology patient, particularly since many women are required to be in "stirrups" at some point in their lives? While little flesh is actually revealed as Bujold plays the part of Claire, the role of the gynecology patient is likened to that of a porn role, a role that could mar the reputation of the performer with whom it is associated. Not only does Bujold portray a gynecology patient, but she portrays a character who appears to be comfortable with her position as patient.

Through her sexual activities with the twins, the narrative suggests that she even enjoys being the object of examination. Thus, because of her perverse pleasures and latent, taboo gratifications, the character of Claire, regardless of her degree of dress, has inevitable risky overtones, that to some are riskier than roles that require the display of more skin.

Given the information that the role of Claire was considered risky by numerous actresses, Claire's comment that she needs "the humiliation as well as the money" is strangely telling. Is the viewer being told that the actress *portraying* the actress also "needs" the humiliation and money? This scene asks the question of what "kind" of woman would allow herself to perform the roles of actress and gyne patient at the levels of both the film's narrative and production. As was suggested through an investigation of the role of the gynecology teaching associate in chapter 3, even within the medical institution the performance of the role of gyne patient is a risky one that threatens to damage the "reputation" of the performer inhabiting such a pornographically overdetermined position.

Claire humiliates herself by mentioning her reproductive organs during lunch at a fancy restaurant. Here the humiliation an actress submits herself to by appearing in the public eye and working within the film industry is narratively equated to the humiliation a patient endures when submitting to the probing gynecologist's eye. Both actress and patient are provoking this humiliation simply by allowing and even promoting themselves as objects of the gaze. Further humiliation occurs when the actress publicly discusses her very private female parts and problems. What happens within clinic walls between doctor and patient is considered private. When Claire discusses her condition in a public setting, the public role of actress becomes confused and conflated with the allegedly private performance of the gyne patient, a seemingly distasteful and inappropriate mix.

Why is the character Claire, the "mutant" woman who triggers the twins' self-destruction, assigned the occupation of actress? The production information for *Dead Ringers* provides Cronenberg's reasoning for this decision: "For Cronenberg, it was important that this character be an actress. 'She's written as an actress because one of the things that the film is about is identity and individuality,' he explains. 'Although I normally steer away from film references, I thought that making this character an actress, who is of course accustomed to playing different roles and slipping in and out of different characters, would work very well for the film.'"[13] By assigning Claire such a profession, Cronenberg makes other meanings here—meanings that exceed issues of "identity and individuality." The choice to make Claire an actress allies an overdetermined performative femininity with pathology. As has been discussed throughout these chapters, the female spectacle in medicine has been systematically "treated" as pathological, due in part to her public performative outbreaks as well as her mysterious, private anatomy. Numerous feminist film theorists claim that the same has been true of female spectacles in mainstream cinema. In the single character of Claire, we have the meeting of the classic cinematic and medical feminines; she has the invisible, internal pathology that makes her a mutant woman, and the pathology of performative femininity that allows her to humiliate herself as actress and public spectacle.[14] For Cronenberg, this mix is inherently volatile. As in his other feminine creations, pathological, anatomical exceptions, whether born or made that way, result not only in public humiliation but often in deadly destruction.

PENILE VAGINA

While subject to male observation and diagnosis within the film narrative, Cronenberg's mutant female creations are also highly dangerous. In Cronenberg's *Rabid*, porn star Marilyn Chambers plays Rose, a woman who has contracted a rabieslike infection after a medical mishap at the Keloid clinic and begins to infect those around her. Transmission occurs when Rose embraces her prey and a phallic-shaped growth becomes erect through a vaginal wound in her armpit, penetrating the unsuspecting victim. As in vampire mythology, the punctured victims in turn become hungry for blood and find victims of their own. They do not grow a fancy armpit-penetrator like Rose, rather they must use the old-fashioned method of maiming and mutilating with their hands in order to cannibalize their victims. Single-handedly, Rose almost succeeds in the complete annihilation of the people of Montreal. However, due to efficient city officials and Rose's self-imposed destruction, the epidemic is controlled.

At the start of the film, Rose is portrayed as a sexually desiring biker chick. After her operation and newfound hunger, she craves victims as though she had an uncontrollable sex drive. Her hunger is insatiable. Chambers portrays Rose in a style reminiscent of a porn performance. However, Rose is not only the delirious, abused, and excessively sexual temptress of porn lore, but is simultaneously the rapist who penetrates victims over and over again until they are left unconscious. In *Rabid*, Chambers, a woman who regularly offers herself as spectacle, in this case not just within the film's narrative but as the well-known star of numerous porn films, portrays a character who is physiologically pathologized and threatening. As in the character Claire, in Rose physiological anomaly commingles with female performativity. Rose is threatening not due to any lack, but due to an excess, one that remarkably resembles and behaves like a penis. In her armpit, where there is normally found smooth skin covered in axillary hair, much like images of the female pudenda, the viewer finds a phallic protrusion, and a lethal one at that. Thus the terror this situation plays upon is one in which a lack is expected and a penis is found. This is a very different scenario than the one Freud proposes in "Medusa's Head." In the case of Rose, woman is not "a being who frightens and repels because she is castrated,"[15] but a being who frightens because she is *not* castrated, because there's something where nothing should be.[16] And that something reminds the male viewer that Rose could indeed be the castrator, stealing his precious weapon for her own violent purposes.

Is Claire's relationship with the twin gynecologists in *Dead Ringers* similar to Rose's with her victims? Certainly Freudian psychoanalysis would insist upon the problematic role of gynecologists because they are continuously faced with vulvas, the lacking wounds that signify castration.[17] But Claire's pathology, like Rose's, also manifests itself in her physiological and phallic-shaped grotesqueness—her three cervixes. While she cannot penetrate with her excesses, they are indeed met "head to head" when she is sexually penetrated. Claire's pathology is not premised on a lack, but on a phallicized abundance. By enlisting psychoanalysis one might be able to explain away such an excess as simply an excessive absence. But there is *something* there. Something frightening and mysterious.

During the opening credits for *Dead Ringers*, Cronenberg uses numerous sixteenth-century medical illustrations: tools for dissection, a woman sitting on a pedestal with flaps of her abdominal fascia splayed open displaying reproductive organs intact, mythological Siamese twin hermaphrodites, twin fetuses in vitro. One particularly interesting drawing shows "The female organs of generation from Jacob Rueff, *Habammenbuch* (1583), which appeared in English as the widely plagiarized and popular *The Expert Midwife* (1637). The anterior wall of the uterus has been dissected to reveal a fetus in vitro. The vaginal canal and the external genitalia exemplify the 'penile vagina'" (see Figure 32).[18] In *The Making of Sex: Body and Gender from the Greeks to Freud*, Thomas Laqueur enlists this same image to illustrate that from classical antiquity to the end of the seventeenth century the prevailing notion of sex was not the two-sex model of sexual difference subscribed to now, but rather one premised on sexual sameness, a sameness alluding to the canonical male body in which "the vagina and external structures are imagined as one giant foreskin of the female interior penis whose glans is the domelike apex of the 'neck of the womb' [or cervix]."[19] In this configuration of sexual difference, men and women are not two sexes. Rather they share the same equipment. On men it is located on the outside of the body, and on women it is found inside the body. And indeed, in the drawing it is clear how the female vagina and uterus are made to represent the male penis and testicles.

I do not wish to imply that Cronenberg or his audience is necessarily familiar

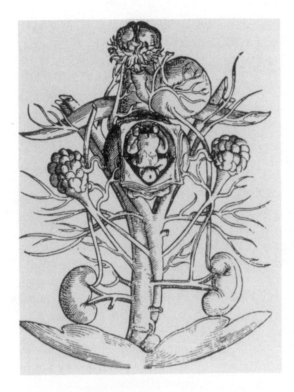

Figure 32. "The female
organs of generation
from Jacob Rueff,
Habammenbuch (1583)."

with the one-sex model that is referenced during his opening credits; rather I focus on this idea in order to complicate notions of Freudian lack and as a means of providing alternative readings of the horror of this film.[20] For centuries before Freud there were other ways in the Western world of imagining female bodies, ways that did not rely on difference as much as sameness. These alternatives did not necessarily work toward a more powerful position for women in society. Instead of being inferior because women were the *opposite* of men, women were seen as lesser because their analogous anatomy was *interior*. Galen, a second-century anatomist, proposed that women were inferior and had less heat than men and thus their "male" organs existed within the body so that they could be warm. While neither view—woman as inferiorly interior or hopelessly lacking—is particularly optimistic with regard to societal attitudes toward women since both consider the female body to be abnormal in relation to the normal male body, they are two different ways of considering female reproductive organs.

Thus Cronenberg, in the tradition of other cultural producers before him, has created two characters, Claire and Rose, who can be viewed as not lacking a penis, but as having phallic-shaped excesses of their own. Then it becomes necessary to ask why women with pathological phalluses become threatening forces in these two films. This is not a threat that may be explained away by necessarily employing the notion of castration anxiety, unless these male spectators have so bought into Lacanian notions of lack that these women are scary because they lack that very lack. Where a lack was expected none was found.[21]

Could Claire and Rose be constructions of what Luce Irigaray had in mind when she titled her work *This Sex Which Is Not One* ? In the case of Claire, she, like other women, is not *one*; she does not have a single, recognized sex organ, namely a penis. Nor is she *two*, though she has the two lips that characterize female genitalia for Irigaray. Rather Claire is unique because she is *three*. Externally, she may appear to have no more than the anticipated *horror of nothing to see*, the hole, that which signifies a lack or absence of male genitalia (given our current two-sex model).[22] But internally, she contains an excess, an excess in the form of three phallacized "necks" of her womb, that render her infertile or neuter—a third term, a tripleness in excess of the twin's doubleness. Cronenberg has created his monster mutant Claire as a frustrated freak of nature. She is an object of sexual and scientific curiosity for the twins rather than, for instance, a woman interjected into their lives in order to force them to question their fear of and hatred toward women. Irigaray's political strategy in replacing female absence with an unlocatable multiplicity does not anticipate the twins' fetishization of the abnormalities of Claire's (un)reproductive organs. In Cronenberg's creations, anatomical multiplicity is simply another difference to be pathologized.

HYSTERIA

Claire is not the only one of Cronenberg's female creations whose medical abnormality is reproductively related. Whereas Claire's pathological excess resides in her uterus, its many chambers and entrances causing her sterility, Nola, in *The Brood* (1979), has a different type of womb-anly problem. Nola is a woman undergoing intense therapy under the supervision of Dr. Raglan. Raglan's specialty is psychoplasmics, "the treatment of serious mental disorder through its physical manifestation in the body."[23] Dr. Raglan's prize patient, Nola, has a "physical manifestation" unlike any he's ever seen. She has, in a sense, become a human uterus, with placental pouches sprouting from various parts of the outside of her body. From the sacks she births tiny deformed children by biting open the pouches and licking away the afterbirth like an animal. These "children of her rage" employ their superhuman strength to brutally murder, over the course of the film, Nola's mother and father and her daughter's schoolteacher, whom Nola suspects of having adulterous thoughts about her husband. Dr. Raglan keeps Nola and the kids locked up at his Somafree Institute and only discovers toward the end of the film that the brood members simply break out of their shed in order to satisfy Nola's angry wishes.

In *The Brood*, like *Dead Ringers*, there is a central female spectacle who is pathologized. She is viewed by her doctor as well as the film audience. Her physiological pathology is intertwined with her emotional weakness. In Nola's case, unlike Claire's, we are instructed that emotional instability both precedes and produces physiological anomaly. In Claire's case, her abnormal uterus most likely preceded and possibly caused an abnormally abundant sexuality. Regardless of the order of events, both women's pathology manifests itself in an inordinate amount of uterus. The more uterus or *hysterus*, the more hysterical. In this sense, Nola and Claire are science-fictive hysterics. Like the classically defined hysteric, they are white, overly emotional women with economic means who do not properly perform their prescribed roles. Simply being a dissatisfied woman, particularly a white dissatisfied woman of means, provides the ingredients for hysteria. The famed nineteenth-century physician Breuer concluded that the hysteria his patient Anna O. displayed was "a 'creative' escape from the boredom and futility of her daily life."[24] However, Nola's and Claire's hysterias take on strange new forms and physiological manifestations. While medical literature has noted women with two cervixes (bifurcates), the trifurcate is a speculative improbability. Similarly, a woman whose psyche allows her to sprout a brood is physiologically impossible. However, both of Cronenberg's anatomical fabrications feed upon deep cultural fantasies regarding the hysteric and her uterine abnormalities. Like classic hysterics, both women are "acting out." Once again, female performativity becomes enmeshed with pathology. Nola especially could be viewed as a classic nineteenth-century hysteric with whom "mental pathology was suppressed rebellion." But with Nola, such performative rebellion is dangerous because, with the tools Raglan has provided, her anger is no longer simply affecting her own body. Rather her performative outbreaks have deadly outcomes for others as well.

The theatricality of psychoplasmics is illustrated in the opening scene of *The Brood*. Dr. Raglan sits on the floor of a proscenium stage facing a white male patient. The auditorium is filled with intrigued spectators. In an eerie psychodrama, Raglan performs many roles within the patient's life, while the male patient interacts, portraying himself, expressing his feelings. At the climax of the performance, the patient rips open his shirt, revealing the fruits of his emotional labor: numerous welts and tissues that have formed on his back and chest due to the psychodrama he and Raglan have just performed. The lights black out, the curtain drops, the spectators file out, "oohing" with amazement. Because this is the first scene of the film, the cinematic spectator is left unsure as to whether he or she has just witnessed a representation of a fictional or a "real" performance within the film's narrative.

It quickly becomes clear that Raglan, through similar psychodramas, is able to aid his patients in bodily alteration. Bodily performativity, Charcot's evidence of hysterical illness, is Raglan's measure of therapeutic success. While men, such as Raglan's male patient, may engage in spectacular bodily performance, naturally it is a woman who is Raglan's most accomplished patient. Nola's production of deformed, homicidal children outperforms the male patient's meager presentation of sores and blisters. In both *Dead Ringers* and *The Brood*, "acting" is framed as a pathological pastime and preoccupation, one that is most often ascribed to and successfully executed by women. Claire, by virtue of her profession, is seen as continuously "acting." As Elliot says to Beverly: "She's an actress, Bev. She's a flake. Plays games all the time. You never know who she really is." Freud connects hysteria to a sort of acting out. In his writings on hysteria, one might think he is writing specifically about the actress: "hysterical movements are always performed with an elegance and co-ordination ... The third, *hallucinatory*, phase of a hysterical attack, the '*attitudes passionnelles*,' is distinguished by attitudes and gestures which belong to scenes of passionate movement, which the patient hallucinates and often accompanies with the corresponding words."[25] Freud notes that hysteria does occur in men, but much more rarely than in women (he put the ratio as about one to twenty). He offers this connection between the female life cycle and hysteria: "As is well known, an early age, from fifteen onwards, is the period at which the hysterical neurosis most usually shows itself actively in females ... The first years of happy marriage interrupt the illness as a rule; when marital relations become cooler and repeated births have brought exhaustion, the neurosis re-appears ..."[26] Nola's and Claire's hysterias take on variant forms. Nola suffers from a cooled marriage and is practically a parody of Freud's notion of the hysteric woman exhausted from "repeated births." Claire, on the other hand, has no happy marriage to relieve her of this malady, nor do her many sexual encounters result in a healing bundle due to her infertility.

Rather Claire's hysteria takes the form of a self-diagnosed psychosexual pain, which in turn causes her to make a further spectacle of herself by sleeping with scores of men. The trope of the oversexed gyne patient from J. Marion Sims's days recurs (see chapter 2). However, the fact that Claire is a white, economically independent woman and not a poor woman of color is an important facet of the film's narrative. Not only have monied white women been the group most often associated with hysteria throughout the history of psychiatry, but they are also the group most associated with fertility specialists. As noted in chapter 2, since the abolition of slavery, white women's reproductivity has been systematically valued over the reproductivity of poor women of color. Sims's medical career mirrors this value shift: his early vesico-vaginal fistula operations focused on slave women and their reproductive capacity; his work after the abolition of slavery focused on white women, particularly wealthy white women and their reproductivity. In this sense, the fictional twin physicians of *Dead Ringers* and their white patient, Claire, fit into a larger tradition established by Sims's early experimentation.

This historical trope of the gynecology patient as an oversexed slave and the male physician as controlling force is narratively played out when Claire is shown in medical gown, restrained in S&M fashion by medical tubing and clamps, with Elliot sexually "examining" her body. Just as the slave woman's body was coded as pathological in order to legitimate the ways in which her body was used, Claire's pathology serves as an explanatory narrative for her complicity in her medical "treatment." In Claire's case, an excessive uterus is linked to excessive female sexuality, which may only be "cured" through the healing powers of patriarchically procured old-fashioned orgasms. Claire voices the success of her "examination" by exclaiming after a heightened climax, "God, Doctor, you've cured me."

One need not subscribe to Freud in order to note the medical institution's assertion of the connection between female sexuality, the uterus, and performative outbreaks. In an article on the medical treatment of Victorian women, Mary Poovey notes how one doctor invoked a theatrical metaphor when describing hysterics: "'These hysteria patients are veritable actresses,' complained Jules Pairet; 'they do not know of a greater pleasure than to deceive. In one word, the life of the hysteric is nothing but one perpetual falsehood; they affect the airs of piety and devotion and let themselves be taken for saints while at the same time secretly abandoning themselves to the most shameful actions.'"[27] Pairet's warning resembles that of the character Elliot's when he cautions Beverly about Claire's flaky game-playing. Multiple role-playing, the very reason Cronenberg states he assigned Claire the profession of actress, is one of the performative pathologies ascribed to the hysteric. This discussion of hysteria and the medical profession is not as historically or theoretically distant as it may seem. Women patients are still often made to feel as though they are "acting out" if they have a pain or illness and are "treated" with a referral to a psychiatrist. Whether "hypochondria" or "hysteria," illness continues to be attributed to femaleness.[28]

Cronenberg's characters, Claire and Nola, represent various ideas about the hysteric: numerous interplays between anomalous reproductive organs, acting out, emotional problems, and femininity. Cronenberg is the cinematic surgeon who fetishizes female pathology, ensuring its isolation and display. And what (Dr.) Cronenberg, who incidentally titled *Dead Ringer*'s production company Mantle Clinic II, Ltd., reasserts throughout many of his films is the inextricability and inevitability of the female body's relation to pathological anatomy and performativity. The closing shot of *The Brood* encapsulates this idea. The camera zooms in on the arm of Nola's daughter, Candice. On her arm is a small lesion, a foreshadowing of the pouch for the "children of her rage" that she will someday bear. There is a sickness out there, and all girls have it.

Mutant Anatomy as Invisible Fetish

Continually, the viewer of *Dead Ringers* may learn about female anatomy only through the twins, who are the sole inspectors of the various women who frequent their exam tables. In the case of Claire's insides, her mysterious vaginal "vault" holds secrets that reach the filmgoer's eyes and ears only through the interpretive lens of the twin physicians. In practices discussed in previous chapters, the exposure of female anatomy for the viewing audience is mandatory. For instance, in Annie Sprinkle's "Public Cervix Announcement" and in gynecological textbooks it is necessary that viewers "see for themselves." In *Dead Ringers*, however, genitalia never enter the camera's frame, maintaining the idea that the on-screen physicians have sole viewing rights (while assuring the fact that *Dead Ringers* will not be rated as pornographic). Likewise, we are shown no visual evidence of Claire's unusual reproductive organs—no ultrasound image or videotape—and must take the twins' word for it. The invisibility of Claire's anatomy adds to its mystery and monstrousness. But the invisibility of the twins' patients' anatomy serves another purpose as well. It allows for Beverly's perception of his patients' anatomy to shift over the course of the film. At the beginning of the film Claire is the only mutant woman and her anomalous pathology makes her special and beautiful; by the end, Claire and *all* women are mutants simply by virtue of being female. All of their deranged insides are both repulsive and in need of medical intervention.

Claire's anomalous uterus initially provokes fascination in the twins. As mentioned earlier in this chapter, when Elliot, posing as Beverly, initially meets Claire's internal anatomy, he welcomes the astounding finding with excitement. Following a bimanual examination in which he has palpated Claire's internal Cerebrus, Elliot mumbles, "That's fantastic" as he withdraws his fingers. He then professes, "I've often thought there should be beauty contests for the inside of the body." Claire replies, both confused and flattered, "I've never had anybody say that about the inside of my body before." To Elliot, Claire's insides are beautiful because they are pathological, rare anomalies rather than the normal-appearing anatomy he usually encounters.

Beverly, too, is initially attracted to Claire's pathology. He falls for Claire, wanting to keep his experiences with her from his brother, thus creating a rift between the twins. When Claire leaves town for a shoot, Beverly is devastated and calls her hotel room to speak with her. Claire is having a meeting with coworkers in her room and her male assistant answers the phone. Believing Claire is being unfaithful to him, Beverly reveals her secret to the assistant: "Have you examined her yet? Do you know she's a trifurcate . . . you might have to classify that as a mutant . . . You have been fucking a mutant." Beverly offers a description of Claire's pathology as a repellent against her suspected lover's advances and in effect conflates the roles of physician and lover by asking whether he has "examined her yet."[29] These various scenes illustrate the ways in which the roles of male heterosexual lover and physician become conflated in *Dead Ringers*: the sexualized role of the physician admires the beauty of his patient's anatomy, and the medicalized role of the lover demands that he understand the physiological state of his love object. Throughout the conflation of these roles, there is a shifting sense of Claire's anatomy; what is initially considered an attractive anomaly becomes a mutant and repulsive deformity.

The fact that the twins are both intrigued and horrified by Claire's anatomy is a symptom of the practice of fetishizing pathology in Western medicine. As noted in the discussion of gynecology textbooks in chapter 4, photographs in these textbooks often depict extreme and even rare cases of various pathologies. In keeping with these images, Claire's anomalous anatomy is the kind of freakish, extraordinary pathology for which physicians like Beverly and Elliot have been waiting. However, Claire's extraordinary pathology, a uterus with three chambers, is particularly meaningful to the physicians because they are twins. Her tripleness is in excess of the twins' doubleness. As Mary Russo notes, Claire, like the twins, is grotesque. Both categories, the male twin and the mutant woman, are "staples of the iconography of the grotesque."[30] And therein lies the source of Claire's beauty and repulsion. The twins identify with Claire, with her multiplicitous abnormality that mirrors and even exceeds theirs.

While the spectacle of the twins is a continual reminder of their doubleness, the film spectator does not view Claire's tripleness. Instead, we are reminded of her tripleness by the visual presence of the tools intended to be used on mutant women like her. These tools are visible throughout the course of the film, creating terrific spectatorial tension. Narratively, the creation of tools boosts the twin's medical career. Their invention of the Mantle retractor brings them awards and prestige early in their medical careers. While the retractor itself is a large, viselike device, Beverly's later inventions, the gynecological instruments for mutant women, take on even more spectacular and horrifying forms. One may make the claim, as Barbara Creed does, that the gynecological instruments for mutant women serve as the fetish replacement for the lackless vulva.[31] It is possible, however, that these tools are the fetish stand-ins for the fetishized internal pathology. The instruments potentially allow the physicians to better visualize or manipulate the other fetish, the mutant female anatomy. Cronenberg's twins cinematically extend the premise established by Sims, the Father of Gynecology, that female reproductive organs are suitable places for medical intervention and require continuous technological innovation for their proper management. While no visible evidence of pathology is provided, the twins' tools stand in as visible evidence of the extent to which the twins must go in order to examine and "treat" such pathology.

Beverly's attitude toward his patients' bodies begins to alter after suspecting Claire of having an affair. His treatment of them changes as a result. Due to his psychological deterioration, even anatomically "normal" women become subject to his tools. When Elliot reprimands Beverly for using the Mantle retractor on a conscious patient, since they invented it expressly for use on anesthetized women, Beverly responds, "There's nothing the matter with the instrument, it's the body, the woman's body was all wrong." Beverly begins to see all women as mutants and in accordance with his new beliefs he creates new tools: "I've been trying to tell you, Eli, you just don't know the kind of patients we've been getting lately. The patients are getting strange. They look all right on the outside, but their insides are deformed. Well I had to deal with it somehow. Radical technology was required." To Beverly, all women are mutant women. Their outsides are normal (normally lacking a penis), but their insides are deformed. And since their insides are not readily visible, it is difficult to know what is hidden there unless one has the proper tools. In every woman Beverly sees Claire, who appears normal on the outside but is deformed on the inside. What is anatomically normal has become pathologized; the instruments are right, the woman is all wrong. Imaginary pathology is Beverly's new obsession, and his tools become the radical technology with which to treat it. Medical intervention is required for all women because all women are deformed.

However, such intervention is never actualized. Although Beverly does bring his tools into surgery, he never succeeds in using them on women. Instead, at the end of the film he uses them on Elliot. The gynecological instruments for mutant women become instruments for separating twins, feeding on the twins' fantasies that they were not simply identical, but actually Siamese twins because of their intertwined psyches. Locked in their apartment, the twins enter a drug stupor and have a regressive birthday party. Eventually, Beverly operates on Elliot with the tools, killing him. Upon waking and finding Elliot's corpse, Beverly leaves the apartment briefly in an attempt to phone Claire. When he hears her voice, he hangs up and returns to the apartment and his own death. The fact that these instruments intended for work on mutant women actually get used on Elliot confirms the fact that both of the twins identify with their women patients; all share the position of grotesque anomalies in "need" of medical intervention. As with Claire, the twins' multiplicity is intolerable and must be rectified with the proper tools. In the case of the twins, the only possible "treatment" for their multiplicity is death.

Real Life Scientific Fiction

For legal reasons, Cronenberg chose not to indicate that *Dead Ringers* was based on a true story. Instead, he bought the rights to the book *Twins*, which was loosely based on the real-life Marcus twins. The Marcus twins were identical twin male gynecologists who were found naked, dead, and emaciated from drug use in a littered apartment. Through autopsies it was found that one twin had been dead days before the other died. It was also discovered that the twins had been evading various malpractice accusations. The story of the Marcus twins gained much national press. They were written about in scores of newspapers and in magazines such as *Esquire*, *Ms.*, and *Harper's*. Cronenberg, fascinated by this real-life foundation for a horror story, helped to write a script that created a fictional account leading up to the twins' real-life demise.

The fact that *Dead Ringers* is based on a true story is at the foundation of the disavowal of its fictionality, helping foster the "scientific" undertone of Cronenberg's "experiment." Harkening back to Benjamin's aspirations for film as a medium that would be fit for representing both art and science, *Dead Ringers* narratively addresses art-science distinctions throughout. For instance, questions of "art" versus "science" arise when Beverly brings his sketches of radical gynecological tools to Anders Wolleck, a metalworker who owns an art gallery. Wolleck is fascinated by Beverly's sketches of the tools:

Wolleck: What are they?
Beverly: They're gynecological instruments for working on mutant women.
Wolleck: Mutant women, that's a great theme for a show.
Beverly: It's not art, I'm a doctor. I need them for my work.

Wolleck does make copies of the tools for himself, which become his own show in the gallery, thus turning Beverly's medical objects into art objects. Although the viewing subject is watching a film, a piece of "art," the narrative of the film points to the notion that "art" is not the issue here. Rather, (Dr.) Cronenberg might have the viewers believe that they are being presented with a piece of "science."

Likewise, in displaying the twin physicians' fascination with and fetishization of the grotesque pathology of the female body, Cronenberg may be seen as offering a critique of the medical and film institutions that condone misogynist behavior. One particular scene offers a possible and pointed critique. When Elliot visits Claire in her "on-location" dressing trailer, she is in the middle of having makeup applied. At the start of the scene, Claire sits in profile. The camera concentrates on only one side of Claire's face. The makeup artist's work is concentrated on the other side of her face and is out of the shot's reach. Elliot, however can see what is being done and is fascinated:

> Claire: I didn't know you were into art.
> Elliot: I'm interested in glamour, the art of glamour.
> Claire: Well, here it is.

Claire turns her head as she and Elliot continue speaking and the makeup artist's work is revealed. Claire has been made up to look as though she has been beaten; she has brownish-blue scabs at her left eye and the left corner of her mouth. For the remainder of this scene, the camera stays focused on the left side of Claire's face—the "punished" side—and the untouched right side is out of the camera's view. Elliot has been fascinated by this artful injury. Claire implies, with her sarcastic "Well, here it is," that the glamour the movie industry has to offer this actress, if not most actresses, is the glamour of portraying the object of violence and abuse. Not only does this scene appear to critique the medical profession with the twin's fascination in the representation of pain, but it also appears to directly comment on the film industry, an industry in which an actress is subjected to endless narrative punishments. In this scene, the artifice of the ideological underpinnings of these two institutions is highlighted. But as the constructedness of the medical and film worlds is pointed to, the film narrative is simultaneously disavowing the fact that *this* film is also constructed, a fiction. Just as Cronenberg is introduced and legitimized by a real-life "Dr." in *Cronenberg on Cronenberg*, the spectator of *Dead Ringers* is somehow supposed to recognize the artifice of the twins' (the medical) and movie business's (the filmic) treatment of Claire without critiquing her narrative treatment within *this* film.

Certainly, the interchanges such as those between Beverly and Wolleck and those between Claire and Elliot could be considered critiques of the worlds of art and science that for centuries have shared the common theme of "mutant women." However, Cronenberg the scientist and artist creating this film has also chosen the same theme for *his* show. Although his film appears to be critiquing or "making fun" of the medical and art institutions that choose the "mutant woman" as their theme, he unself-consciously reiterates this notion in his construction of Claire and his employment of gynecology as metaphor for "the mind-body split." While he is critical of the represented artistic and medical worlds found in his film, Cronenberg remains uncritical of his own representational practice.[32] Perhaps he has been caught up in what Joan Copjec terms "the delirium of clinical perfection"[33] in that Cronenberg the film practitioner has usurped a clinical gaze in order to engage in the creation of his science experiment, *Dead Ringers*. Harkening back to Sims, Cronenberg's employment of scientific metaphor may be seen as an excuse for ideologically and teleologically free experimentation.

Cronenberg himself offers one question that fuels his experimentation, a question mimicked in the film almost word-for-word by Elliot: "I'm really saying that the inside of the body must have a completely different aesthetic. You take the most beautiful woman in the world, and you cut her open—is she as beautiful on the inside?"[34] Given this sentiment, that the insides of a female body have a different aesthetic economy than the outsides, the tools for mutant women, designed by Cronenberg himself, are the realization or externalization of that interior aesthetic. The tools are like metal casts of Beverly's and Cronenberg's twisted fantasy of (pathologized) vaginal beauty.

In Cronenberg's statement, it also becomes clear that he is fascinated by the precise issues of sameness and difference that fueled Sims's experimentation on slave women. Compatibility between insides and outsides are the question here. For Sims, the incompatibility of outsides (racial difference) legitimized surgical experiments based on internal similarities (anatomical sameness). Cronenberg enlists surgical speculation to question the compatibility of external aesthetic beauty with internal beauty. Regardless of the nature of Cronenberg's aesthetic quandary, his question does not entertain the politics of "cutting women open." In contemporary film this "cutting women open" has traditionally meant the frequent display of the maiming, raping, and brutalizing of female bodies. In medicine, "cutting women open" has been overused as a technique for "treating" women (e.g., surgical procedures such as clitoridectomy, oopherectomy, or removing ovaries, hysterectomy, sterilization, etc.). Cronenberg, not unlike the Father of Gynecology, assumes that a surgeon, cinematic or otherwise, should not be held responsible for the deeper meanings of his brilliant experiments.

Within the narrative, Cronenberg addresses the medical world's "treatment" of women, specifically wealthy white women. He presents an undeniably ironic scene in which Elliot professes to a group of medical students that the physician's relationship to his patient combines "compassionate curiosity with social responsibility." The viewer is shown the deluded patient who clutches Beverly's arm and says, "It's hard to find someone in the medical profession you can trust. I trust you." The viewer witnesses the completely inappropriate way in which the Mantle twins run their practice and lives. The spectator watches Elliot confide to Beverly: "The beauty of our business is you don't have to get out much to meet beautiful women." Such words undoubtedly position the sacrosanct medical sphere as badly tarnished. *Dead Ringers* could seem to be a critical film because it narratively questions the medical practice of two acclaimed and wealthy white male physicians. But these scenes function less as a critique of misogynist medicine and more as an elaboration of the theatricality of gynecology that Cronenberg finds to be such a perfect metaphor for the mind-body split.[35] And this metaphor, as noted above, is both race- and gender-specific.

The fact that these twin physicians are male gynecologists is an integral part of this filmic equation. Male gynecologists have both sets of tools: penis (phallus) and metal instruments (speculum, Mantle retractor, tools for mutant women, etc.). Thus they are doubly powerful. Imagine a similar film about twin female urologists: the film would indeed be radically altered and differently inflected. Gynecology was not a random choice. In gynecology, women and their genitals occupy the sole position of patient and spectacle; in *Dead Ringers*, horror and titillation are represented as gynecology's inseparable and inevitable components. Likewise, the twin fertility specialists work entirely on wealthy white women. How might this film have functioned differently if the twins used their tools on poor women of color in a public hospital? Once again, the film would be radically altered.

Dead Ringers' representation of gynecology, which plays upon the abuse and pathological nature of the female body and the fetishization of female pathology, mirrors actual instances of gynecological practice, invoking some of the real-life terrors associated with this area of medicine. Television and the popular press capitalize on these horrors. The serial *Law and Order* presents the docudrama of the gynecologist who sexually abused his patients. Newspapers and magazines expose Dr. Burt, who surgically altered his patients' vulvas without their knowledge or consent so there would be more clitoral contact during intercourse. The reason gynecological horror is newsbreaking material is that gynecology itself is an overdetermined practice, laden with an array of power and gender-based connotations that signify terror and eroticism. Thus *Dead Ringers*, textually and in its production, shares some of the gynecological practice's underlying and naturalized premises: men want to understand and dissect women, women are pathologized spectacles, and so on. In other words, this representation, *Dead Ringers*, is itself a product of gynecological practice. However, *Dead Ringers* is simultaneously productive. It asserts, among other things, the erotics and terror of gynecological practice in revised and horrifying ways. Thus we may consider this film to be simultaneously symptomatic and productive, feeding on cultural knowledge about gynecology and female bodies while creating a new pool of images and ideas for a mass audience.[36] These new meanings help to further define gynecological practice, clarifying and picturing some of its unspoken terrors.

Surgeon-Spectator

I heard about *Dead Ringers* for years before I finally ventured to view it. I had avoided the film because I knew it was about gynecologists engaging in questionable practices, I was familiar with Cronenberg's brand of psychological horror, and I was afraid of being terrorized by it. After viewing the film, I was deeply disturbed for days. Only with multiple viewings could I find more "distance" from the film. But a very peculiar thing happened. I found as I mentioned the film to women I knew, including film scholars, that a great number of them expressed feelings I had had before viewing *Dead Ringers*—they had heard about the film, were aware of the subject matter and even the story line, and had refused to view it. Of course there are women who choose to view *Dead Ringers* and find pleasure in its perverse practices. But although there is a wide spectrum of viewing possibilities and positions for women in this film, I was struck by the number of women who told me they knew about the film and had specifically made an effort not to see it.

In his essay "Vile Bodies and Bad Medicine," Pete Boss explores popular ideas about modern medicine found in horror films and theorizes the position of the spectator in this contemporary genre that is riddled with a proliferation of brutally violent images. He briefly considers the notion of spectator as surgeon, referencing Cronenberg's *Rabid* as evidence: "Freed from interest in character we watch Marilyn Chambers' skin graft in *Rabid* (1977) with the detached eye of a surgeon as strips of flesh are peeled away by some kind of electric slicer. It is her flesh which fascinates and appalls us rather than the character's plight—she is reduced to mere tissue."[37] Boss suggests yet another component of the replication of the surgeon-patient relationship found in film, that of viewing subject as surgeon to the projected patient. From Benjamin, we learn that the filmmaker is a surgeon who manipulates and edits the film body at the level of mechanical production. Cronenberg asserts that he is a cinematic surgeon who reorganizes the film's narrative body at the level of production. From Heath, we learn another way in which the film and its filmmaker may suture the viewing subject into the film text, drawing on both narrative and mechanical production at the level of the cinematic apparatus, incorporating a structural notion of the viewing subject. This suggests that the position of the viewing subject is like an organ that the filmmaker adds to the film body, suturing it into place. Boss suggests yet another way in which the idea of a surgeon enters the cinematic apparatus. He claims that the actual viewing subject may be a surgeon. The film itself, specifically Cronenberg's variety of medicalized horror, positions the viewer as surgeon who, in order to witness his brutalizing and violent work consisting of cuts and dismemberment, must distance himself from the body in question.

Such mandatory "distance" is not always possible. Given that there are women who have heard about *Dead Ringers*, are horrified by its premise or subject matter, and refuse to view it, what place does the audience who *refuses* or chooses *not* to view a specific film have in a critical investigation of that film? Is their decision not to view *Dead Ringers* simply a refusal to identify with the vulnerable and pathologized female patients they would see on screen?[38] Or, following Boss's proposal, is it an unwillingness to be positioned as distanced surgeon-spectators? Unlike *Rabid*, there is actually very little bloody, doctor-to-patient violence committed against the female body (I omit from this category of violence S&M-type acts which some critics would claim to be violence against women). We do not witness brutal beatings, rapes, or slashings. But I would contend that for many women gynecology itself rests so precariously on the boundaries of medicine and violence that the mere suggestion that a woman would be made to suffer pain in the exam may be enough to horrify the most assured female spectator.[39] On-screen the instruments for mutant women are not used on women at all. However, their mere visual presence is enough to suggest excruciating cruelty and perversion. Similarly, even a brief description of this film's narrative convinces certain potential viewers that they do not want to view it. Suggestion, given prevalent attitudes toward gynecology, may be more terrifying than the viewing itself.

Certainly *Dead Ringers* need not be widely viewed in order to be productive of new meanings. Through discussion about the film, a mythology has developed surrounding this text that keeps some from viewing it. The same fears that circulate around the practice of gynecology or "going to the gynecologist" may fuel the mythologies surrounding this representation of gynecological practice. In other words, a refusal to view the film may be stirred by the same set of horrors that prevent some women from visiting the gynecologist. They are resisting or rejecting the position of vulnerable subject to a controlling institution, be it medicine or cinema, thereby refusing to accept the role of compliant viewer or cinematic patient. In some ways, this confirms Cronenberg's assertion of himself as cinematic surgeon. As a contemporary auteur, his name is so closely allied with *Dead Ringers* that a refusal to view his film could be considered a refusal to see the doctor. In a very roundabout way, Cronenberg has affirmed his power as physician, his representational practices mirroring gynecological practice in the many ways discussed. The epigraph to this chapter points to this with perverse clarity. Cronenberg is "playing doctor" throughout his films on a variety of levels, reaffirming old knowledge and even producing new and terrifying myths about the female body and gynecology. While "playing doctor," Cronenberg recognizes the problems of the filmic and medical institutions with relation to the pathologized female body. But he has fetishized these pathologies in his film product, making them sexy and terrifying, eroticizing them for the potential spectator.

7 The Other End of the Speculum: Woman-Centered Alternative Practice

Variation

Scripted here are multiple configurations of an alternative, woman-centered pelvic theater. Assembled from a variety of women's experiences and ideas, this speculative fiction is a reflection of past, present, and future practices.[1] This collage of writings is about potential change, about opening up possibilities for a new cast of characters, shifting roles, sets, costumes, and props in the production of gynecology and therefore in the production of female performance.

The practices illustrated in these fictions are indebted to those participants in the women's health movement who, beginning in the 1960s, launched a harsh critique against the styles of practice of the predominantly male medical establishment. They addressed vital issues in women's health, including reproductive rights, sterilization abuse, medical experimentation, informed consent, and the prevalence of often unnecessary and disfiguring surgeries (e.g., hysterectomy).[2] An explicit aspect of their critique was the creation of new practices or alternative pelvic theaters. In the early 1970s, self-help groups formed in which mostly white, middle-class women shared information and stories, educating themselves about their bodies, the medical establishment, and alternative treatments. For some groups, these informal meetings led to the widespread dissemination of information on women's health and options (the Boston Women's Health

Speculative Fiction

From the bus I can see the lettering on the window: The Women's Health Center. "This place is different," my niece, Rita, promised. "It's better." Getting off the bus and crossing the street, I am finding it impossible to prevent that familiar, annual terror. I picture myself in that ridiculous position, feeling like a plucked chicken about to be filleted. But in this dreamy cartoon, the gynecologist-butcher knows I am alive and either pretends I'm not or diverts my attention while deboning me—speaking about the weather, my holiday plans, current events, *anything* but my body.

I enter the building. The center looks more like a home than a clinic: comfortable couches, children's toys, books. The women who work there are wearing street clothes instead of white mice lab coats and it doesn't smell like rubbing alcohol. One woman welcomes me, handing me a chart to fill out. In the well-worn waiting room, I begin detailing my medical history. I fill in the blank with a "12." Twelve. Even though it was so long ago, I remember it like it was yesterday. At twelve I got my period and at thirteen I was raped by this man in his thirties, my cousin's boyfriend. My mother knew but didn't want to talk

Book Collective and their many editions of *Our Bodies, Ourselves* is one of many examples), and for others these gatherings grew into women-controlled, woman-centered alternative clinics (e.g., the Los Angeles Health Center and the Emma Goldman Clinic). The groups began diversifying, broadening their scope of issues so that women with a variety of experiences and backgrounds would be included. New organizations formed, addressing the health concerns of specific groups (e.g., National Black Women's Health Project, Native American Women's Health Education Resource Center, and local groups such as Chicago's Lesbian Community Cancer Project). Access to health care, including the pelvic theater, continues to be an issue of prime concern.

Groups that run woman-centered, alternative clinics often specialize in well-woman health care, an inclusive term that asserts the wellness of the majority of women who seek gynecological care: "Well-woman excludes only the independent management of serious medical or gynecological conditions that require medical or surgical interventions for diagnosis or therapy."[3] The majority of women, therefore, fit within the well-woman category. Nonphysician practitioners are the care providers. They incorporate self-help practices into the exam while encouraging the continuation of these practices outside the clinic but "physician care, when needed, is available on site or by referral."[4] Self-help incorporates a range of practices including but not limited to "alternative" thera-

about it. I think she blamed me for the trouble. She thought she was doing her job by making me an appointment with a gynecologist. I remember my girlfriend, Londa, the morning of my appointment, looking at me as though I were about to die, "Oooh, It's going to hurt a lot!" I was terrified. The next thing I remember I was on my back, my legs spread with this graying man clanking metal instruments around on a tray. He told me that no girl my age should even be thinking about having sex. I should be out playing, not in the bedroom. And then he was examining me, touching me and I was squirming because I was scared and he kept saying, "It doesn't hurt. Stay still. RELAX." But I was so scared I started crying. He just stuck this cold metal thing into me too quickly without any warning and I screamed and he said, "Now that wasn't so bad." Yes it was. I didn't go back to any gynecologist until I was twenty-three and seven months pregnant.

*

She finishes filling out the chart and hands it back to one of the women working. There are fliers papering the waiting room—information about child care, lesbian groups, new contraceptives, and domestic violence. So much information. Shelves of books, some in

pies (e.g., home treatments for vaginal infections, nutritional changes, herbal remedies), regular self-exam (breast, cervical, vaginal, vulvar), menstrual extraction, menstrual diaries, and stress reduction.[5] The term "self-help" is not meant to exclude or diminish the importance of the treatment provided by others than oneself. Rather, self-help is one way of extending the performance from within the exam to include those everyday life performances that promote wellness and prevent or manage illness.

In the alternative pelvic theater, there is an expanded role for the female client. No longer measured against a patient model who is properly passive, receptive, insured, white, thin, and heterosexual, this alternative pelvic theater figures into its blockings and scripts ways of including the female client as an active performer irrespective of her resources and identity. She is invited to participate in the performance regardless of her race and ethnicity, age, weight, abilities and disabilities, sexual practices and identity, class, employment and economic status, educational level, religion, and language abilities. Scripts must not be written based on appearances. A client's needs must not be anticipated, assumed, or dictated given where she falls within the above categories. For example, because a woman is postmenopausal or disabled does not necessarily mean she is disinterested in sexual activity. A graduate degree does not guarantee that a woman knows what or where her cervix is. Because a woman is young and African

Spanish, on women's health care. There's even one called *How to Stay Out of the Gynecologist's Office.* She laughs at the title. She should show it to her school nurse. That's who told her she should come in the first place. A smiling woman who has her chart introduces herself as Sophie, and leads her to a table with chairs in another room. She feels just like she did last week when she was sent to the principal's office. Sophie is genuinely sweet, though, and welcomes her to the clinic, explaining that the health center is a collective of women health workers, physicians, and therapists. The only reason she came at all was because this place is all women. She asks about this contraceptive that they put in your arm. They had pamphlets about it at the nurse's office.

*

So you're not a doctor or a nurse? "No," she explains, looking into my eyes. Hers are unhurried. "As you were told when you made the appointment, I'm a health worker who has been trained in the clinic. Here we believe that women can be trained to do basic well-woman care like pap smears, pelvic exams, infection checks, breast exams." Well-woman. That's true, I'm not sick. Just like I wasn't sick when I had my baby, but being at the hospi-

American does not mean she has multiple sexual partners, is incapable of using a barrier method (diaphragm, cervical cap, or condom), and is heterosexual. Such assumptions riddle conventional gynecological practice. However, because women participate in an alternative practice does not mean they are immune to such stereotypes, biases, and racism. Rather, alternative practitioners must continuously interrogate and battle their own individual assumptions.

An alternative, woman-centered pelvic theater must not position a non-English speaker or a deaf woman who signs or a disabled woman who is unable to get into lithotomy position as a disruptive glitch in an otherwise swift, efficient, and economically productive clinical machine. Nor are the great number of women who have been sexually abused, be they survivors of incest, rape, or assault, considered to be "trouble" patients due to their possible apprehensions regarding examination. There should be no prescribed "proper" female performative response to examination or ideal female perfomer. There should be no standard script or model patient performance. Rather, attention must be focused on the flexibility of the clinic, on the way the clinic can adapt to a client's performance. There needs to be a continuous reassessment of services and practices to assure such accessibility. An alternative clinic must invite the multiplicity of attitudes, subjectivities, and positionalities that women enlist when approaching and confronting gynecology.

tal with all those tubes and monitors and the way the doctors and nurses acted, I certainly was treated like I was diseased, like I was about to give birth to an eight-pound tumor. "We work in a team with midwives, doctors, and other health workers. We've gone through extensive training here at the clinic. If a problem is beyond the scope of our training, then we'd have a client see one of our doctors." I'm not a patient. I'm a client. Presumed well until found otherwise? *There's* a switch. It's just that I've never gone to a place where I didn't see a doctor. That's why I pay a ton of money every month for insurance so I can go anyplace I want. There are no uniforms here. The walls aren't white. They have awful magazines in the waiting room. It makes me a little shaky not seeing a doctor. But it also could be all that coffee I drank this morning. She says that the clinic runs on a self-help philosophy and that I should ask as many questions as I want to and can be as active in the exam as I want to be. Ask questions? Never heard that one in a medical office before.

*

I tell my sister to tell her right off: I don't have any insurance. I don't have any public aid. I just came to the States two weeks ago and I don't have any money. They all seem very

Variation is the rule, rather than the exception. As with the alternative text *New View of a Woman's Body*, discussed in chapter 4, physiologically and anatomically emphasis must be placed on the wide variety of normal—sizes and shapes of labia, breasts, stomachs, hips—rather than on any arbitrary and limiting standard. Body modification, including piercings, tattoos, implants, and plastic surgeries, must also be considered part of that variety. Which leads to a needed problematization of the term "woman-centered." How will the alternative pelvic theater define "woman"? Will there be space for a surgically made woman—a male to female transsexual—in the alternative pelvic theater? What about a surgically made hermaphrodite like Les in *Linda, Les, and Annie*, who looks like a man but who has an intact vulva, vagina, and cervix beneath his constructed penis? Ideally, definitions of "woman" must retain a certain flexibility that the foremothers of the women's health movement might not have anticipated at its inception.

Vision

This alternative pelvic theater provides the client with a multiplicity of choices. Among those choices are multiple treatment options that include alternative or non-Western therapies. Rather than overlooking the examined woman's posi-

nice here, but I know nothing is ever free. My sister tells her what I've said in English. The woman smiles. My sister listens to her answer and then explains to me that the clinic runs on a "suggested donation" basis. At the end of our visit, she will give me an envelope and I put in whatever I can. My donation is anonymous—if I can't donate today, maybe I can next time. Seems impossible. How can this work? I almost didn't come today because I was so afraid they would just tell me to go home even though I have this pain.

*

"A pap smear," I blurt, coolly. That is my answer to Linda asking why I am at the clinic. No problems. Nothing wrong. In the past, I've walked into a pap smear feeling fine. Nothing wrong. But by the time I leave, everything is wrong—having sex is wrong, not having sex is wrong, being a woman is wrong. Linda doesn't bury her head in my chart. We discuss my medical history carefully. She handles my past gently, doesn't rip through it. Her metronome is considerate, paced just right, around a slow trot rather than a roaring gallop. She says we have a whole hour and that if we can't get through everything we can always schedule some more time. She doesn't act like there is something burning in the oven. She

tion as spectator, as is the case in most traditional gynecological practices, a great deal of attention is placed on the woman's experience of the exam and therefore on her role as active performer, decision maker, spectator, and possibly even as self-spectator. If she chooses to do so, the client may use a mirror to observe what the clinician does during the external genital exam and the collection of cervical smears. Likewise, the client is offered the choice of inserting her own speculum and viewing her own cervix, two possibilities commonly excluded from the traditional performance of the pelvic exam. The prop of speculum is no longer metal, but is plastic so that the client may take it home to continue self-exam if she chooses. It is important to note that these practices of self-observation and self-exam are offered as options. A client will not be judged as performing improperly or being noncompliant if she refuses such choices.

Self-spectatorship is virtually unaccounted for within traditional gynecological theater. Self-spectatorship confounds traditional spectator-spectacle gendered power relationships, like those outlined by Laura Mulvey, allowing the woman to embody both spectator and spectacle simultaneously. It could be theorized that the woman thus becomes both "evils," both the "bearer of the look" and the scopophilic voyeur. Instead I would argue that cervical self-exam specifically and self-spectatorship in general offer a critique of Mulvey, representing

asks me if I am currently sexually active. I answer yes and she says, "With men or women or both?" There it is. A question I never expected. "Both," I answer, "Right now, I'm with a woman." Last pap smear, a nurse practitioner went off on me when I told her I wasn't using birth control. She answered snippily, "Do you want to get pregnant?" and launched into a series of statistics. I let her go, my head retracting into my shell. I knew if I told her "I don't need birth control right now. I have sex with a woman" she would have imploded. Linda brings up lesbian safer sex stuff—homemade dental dams, which infections can be spread between women, and so on. Interesting.

*

You didn't ask me if my babies were from different fathers. Or whether I am married to my sexual partner. You didn't assume I am on welfare. You did not tell me—before you even examined me or asked me any questions—that the problem I'm having is from a sexually transmitted disease. You didn't even have that look in your eyes—of disgust or dislike—all because of my skin color. That's what I've gotten before. They're white people dressed in white, everything so white. I've gotten lots of disapproval and not much else.

an almost complete departure from the traditional gynecological and cine-matic apparatuses.

Cervical self-exam is yet another practice indebted to the women's health movement. In the 1960s and '70s all over the United States, women in early self-help groups inserted speculums in order to see their cervixes and vaginas, an opportunity previously reserved for medical professionals. The speculum was an icon of this movement, a symbol of the importance of knowing one's own body, of taking control of and being knowledgeable about patriarchal medicine's tools. However, putting the tool or prop of the speculum in the hands of the woman client is not any guarantee of control, knowledge, or complete agency. The problematic, utopian rhetoric of these early health activist pioneers has led some current theorists to reject the idea of self-spectatorship and self-help altogether as part of the pelvic performance. In her important essay "A Cyborg Manifesto: Science, Technology, and Socialist-Feminism in the Late Twentieth Century," Donna Haraway proclaims the speculum to be an antique symbol in an age when women continually interface with sophisticated technologies: "The speculum served as an icon of women's claiming their bodies in the 1970s; that handcraft tool is inadequate to express our needed body politics in the negotiation of reality in the practices of cyborg reproduction. Self-help is not enough."[6]

*

Jackie is knowledgeable and relaxed so I ask many questions. She answers them. I find myself asking about masturbation, a topic I have never in my forty-eight years brought up at a medical visit. But even though I'm old enough to be her mother she doesn't treat me like a deviant or speak about it so clinically you'd never want to touch yourself again. One question I have about HIV she can't answer. She says so, writes it down, and will find it out in addition to giving me a hotline number. She explains the exam to me from start to finish. Even though she makes it sound easy and relaxed, I hear the fourteen-year-old Londa, "Oooh, it's going to hurt a lot!" Sensing what I thought was well-disguised squeamishness, Jackie lets me know that if at any time during the exam I want her to stop, she will. That simple. I am in charge. She explains that she will, if I want, teach me how to insert my own speculum, the instrument used to view my cervix. Some women find it more comfortable to insert their own. I tell her maybe. Yeah, right. Not likely. After she takes my blood pressure, I follow her to the exam room and she leaves me there to undress from the waist down.

The varied forms of advanced technologies Haraway refers to throughout her essay and the various ways today's female cyborg (woman-machine hybrid) confronts them might be ill-represented by the speculum. But it is surprising that Haraway would be ready to discard the speculum so swiftly and so completely.

While self-help may not be enough given the female cyborg's continual negotiation with new technologies, it may still be a place to start. The speculum or "handcraft tool," as menially mechanical and prepostmodernist as it may be, is still an integral part of the pelvic theater and is often utilized in conjunction with more advanced technologies. Likewise, this used icon, reduced by Haraway to the realm of symbolic inadequacy, continues for many to function as a symbol of the profound tension associated with gynecological exams. As noted by Annie Sprinkle in chapter 5, the simple staged act of revealing a metal speculum provokes many women audience members into vocalizing their anxiety. The speculum does not only function as an icon of 1970s' style empowerment; rather its impact is otherwise symbolic, signifying the pains and stresses of contemporary gynecology, as high-tech as it may be.

In their 1981 *Camera Obscura* article, Stephen Grosz and Bruce McAuley review *Self-Health* and *Healthcaring*, two self-help films made in the mid-1970s.

I look up at the single small window in the exam room. There's still time. Talking has been pleasant, but now . . . I remember, repeating it to myself like a newfound mantra, "Anytime I want to I can just tell her, stop." It is a calming thought. I take a deep breath. I still look around the room, feeling caged in. It's not Jackie, she's a very nice young woman. I just hate this. Is there any oxygen in here? There is the table. The Table. And there are the stirrups. The Stirrups. Just looking at them makes my skin ice. Medieval torture devices disguised as modern medicine. The walls dance with drawings of vaginas with speculums and cervixes, a diagram of diaphragms, a breast-exam illustration, a chart labeled "Cervical Dilation." There are no crinkly paper robes or sheets to cover myself. I take off my pants, then my underwear, and drape them over the arm of a chair. Before, at the doctor's, I would hide my underwear. Place it under the pants so they wouldn't see. I kept them for myself. Not just anybody should be able to see your underwear, especially if they've just been on. Here, I don't cover them. Instead I allow the underwear to sit on top of the pants. Half-dressed. I have my own shirt on. Although I'm naked below, the cotton top feels better than paper. At least I feel like myself. How can any person feel like herself wearing pa-

They maintain that self-help, particularly cervical self-exam, may actually be detrimental because the woman cannot recognize pathology: "we can see the value of sharing basic facts. Yet when a group of women are shown learning to look at the cervix (with the aid of speculum, mirror and flashlight) the importance of this activity is less clear. Moreover, the fact that the cervix shown is abnormal goes virtually unnoticed and raises the important issues of how these women are going to use the observations of self-examination."[7] Certainly self-exam will not replace, nor do its supporters suggest it should replace, a yearly pap smear or other preventative diagnostic testing. Rather the impetus behind self-exam is not necessarily pathology-oriented at all. As an early self-help article attests, "Self-exam stands the medical approach on its head: we observe *well women* in our normal states. We do so not to search out hidden sickness but for its own sake."[8] But are Grosz and McAuley suggesting that a woman should only look at her cervix if she has knowledge about pathology or is attended by somebody who does? Diagnostically, the importance of self-exam, particularly vulvar self-exam, is now recognized by medical professionals. Ideally, by examining her vulva regularly, the patient may detect possible pathology such as lesions and warts.[9] However, because a woman does not have all the tools of self-diagnosis does not mean she should be excluded from the possibility of self-

per? Those backless cloudy cloth gowns aren't any better either. Because of my bad knee and my large size I have trouble getting on the table. Jackie knocks on the door and asks if I need any help. Without a word, she assists me onto the table.

*

This one doctor was recommended to me. He is like one of those baby photographers who holds up the yellow squeaky toy so that the kid forgets what's really happening—the finger triggering the lens. But before I see him, a nurse takes me into the exam room. She asks me two questions and puts me on the table with my feet in the stirrups. Then she leaves. I lie that way for at least fifteen minutes. It seems like forever. I don't have a magazine. Nothing. The muscles in my inner thighs start to shake and I am so cold. The door opens. I see him between my knees. And with an "And how are we today?" he launches into the chat and my crotch, never looking me in the eye once. I can't get a word in. He doesn't tell me anything about what he is doing and I certainly can't see what is going on. At first, I feel it is my job to answer his questions about summer vacation and favorite foods as best I can even though I don't really want to. I want to scream I am so angry. I

spectatorship. Self-spectatorship may precede and even lead to learning, rather than vice versa.

The possibility of self-spectatorship within the pelvic theater becomes all the more important as the medical industry becomes increasingly technologized. Paula A. Treichler and Lisa Cartwright cite Grosz and McAuley's discussion of cervical self-exam in their introduction to *Camera Obscura 28: Imaging Technologies, Inscribing Science* in order to stress that women taking over medical imaging is not the answer: "Yet even as we may resist the medicalizing and marketing of female images, it is not easy to see precisely what would constitute a counternarrative. Surely not the denial to women of knowledge of the medical marketplace. Nor the appropriation by women of medical imaging—a point argued by Stephen Grosz and Bruce McAuley . . . [They] suggest that in ultimately assuming 'that the gaze is an incontrovertible source of knowledge,' both films leave unexamined the potential for reorganizing the health care system, more clearly differentiating dominant medicine from health, and more obviously protecting women from serious danger and risk."[10] Once again, the reasoning here is that self-exam threatens to replace medical exams that will "protect" women from danger and risk. Rather, as illustrated by the speculative fiction, self-exam can potentially increase a woman's participation in her own care and ensure that she continue to receive care. And, as the many practices, projects, and clinics that

have these fantasies of squeezing my muscles really tight so that his fingers or instruments break. Maybe I can picket his office, write a letter to the newspaper. But, you know, I don't do any of these things. I leave my body, leave those chunks of flesh on the table for his inspection, and go for a walk in my head.

*

Evelyn is undressed. Even though the room is warm, she is shaking. The health worker enters the exam room. Evelyn will not meet her gaze. Since the beginning of the visit she has found reasons to look this way and that. She assures the health worker that she wants the exam. She needs the exam. She must go through with the exam. The health worker, sensing her apprehension, reminds her that she can stop the exam whenever she wants. Evelyn raises her voice, "You've told me that!" then lowers it, "I'm fine. Just do it, OK? Please." Evelyn places her socked feet in the footrests and slides down to the end of the table. The health worker places the back of her hand on Evelyn's inner thigh to start the exam. All of Evelyn's muscles tighten, her breathing becomes rapid, she clinches her eyes closed, grimacing as if she is in excruciating pain. The health worker removes her hand.

arose out of the women's health movement illuminate, the practice of cervical self-exam is about larger issues than simply investigating one's own cervix. It *is* about imagining a new kind of health care that organizes the female body and its relationship to health and pathology in new ways and therefore reconfigures issues of power and control. As imaging technologies become more and more sophisticated, the impetus behind the practice of cervical self-exam becomes all the more important. Participation in one's own care is vital in a medical world of escalating technologies, along with the important critical investigation of new technologies such as those contained in Treichler and Cartwright's two edited volumes.

If we must have icons, we should not discard the speculum. Haraway's critique that "self-help is not enough" is well heeded as a substantial amount of self-help literature employs essentializing rhetoric and is saddled with other related problems. However, by suggesting that we discard icons of the 1970s, particularly the speculum, Haraway might involuntarily ally herself with a popular brand of postfeminism, one that suggests that these early activists genitalized women's health care rather than acknowledging the fact that the goals of these early activists are still far from realized. While it is popular to believe that we have moved beyond such icons, these more basic technologies have not been eliminated, but augmented by newer technologies.

Evelyn screams "I'm OK. I'm OK. I'm fine. Just do the exam" and begins sobbing. The health worker helps Evelyn sit up and suggests she get dressed.

*

Linda is back with a steel bowl of warm water. She does not match her surroundings— she's much too kind for speculums and stirrups. I ask her why she does this and she smiles, pleased at my question, describing her long-time commitment to women's health care and how she sees the collective as a way of responding to the way women are often dealt with in medicine.

It is so strange, being naked in a room with a virtual stranger. Here are my legs, my knees, my belly. Linda reaches into a drawer and reveals a plastic speculum. They use plastic so that women can take them home after the exam if they want to be able to see their cervixes. I *will* say that it's much less intimidating than its clanking metal cousin. She asks me if I'd like to insert my own. No thanks, I'll let you do it. OK, she says. No pressure. She shows me how it works anyway. Lets me hold it. I used to think that if I touched a speculum some alarm would go off, that you had to have a variety of letters next to your name

Consider other "older" technologies like the gas engine or the telephone. Just because they were invented years ago does not mean we should refrain from critically considering them, particularly given their widespread use. Likewise, the speculum is a predecessor of new gynecological technologies. Understanding how the speculum organizes the female body and spectatorship within the exam provides clues to understanding new technologies. The speculum is still very much in use and its power as a symbol reflects its power as a tool in actual practice. Instead of discarding the speculum, let us have multiple icons that reflect the range of technologies the cyborg confronts on a daily basis—everything from the lowly handcraft tool to the technologically advanced. Self-help has a place in the technologized space in which we live. The use of the speculum in cervical self-exam may only provide a limited view, what Haraway refers to as a "situated knowledge," but it is one worth having and knowing.[11]

Difference

An alternative pelvic theater emphasizes the multiple array of gazes at play— that the client is as much an active spectator and participant in her exam as the

in order to understand its complexities. After placing my speculum in the warm water, Linda asks me to put my heels in the footrests. Not stirrups, footrests. No accompanying visions of riding horses or of being saddled up. She makes them sound almost comforting. I assume that lovely position. Unfortunately some things never change. But the table back is raised so that I can see Linda's face. She doesn't bury her face between my legs. In the past I've thought, what *are* they doing down there? Linda offers me a hand mirror. "To make sure my hair isn't mussed?" I say in my best girlie voice. Linda laughs. "So you can watch what I'm doing," she says, gathering swabs and slides. I accept the mirror. She puts on her gloves and checks the outside of my vagina, describing what she sees: clitoral hood, clitoris, labia minora and labia majora (the lips), urethra . . . Wait a second. "Yeah that, urethra, that's where I pee out of? Could you show me where it is?" It is embarrassing. Here I am, thirty-four years old and I don't know where I pee out of. Linda separates the inner lips and points to this little puckery opening. I always thought it was higher or inside or something. Actually, the whole view is pretty exceptional, seeing it all—*my* lips, *my* clitoris. I never looked at myself before. That's me. I find I am fascinated by my own

clinician. In addition to the possibility of using a mirror and inserting her own speculum, there is no drape-sheet curtain sectioning front stage from backstage. There is no medical costume, no gown that a woman must exchange for her own clothes. There is no master performer who uses the woman patient as prop. Likewise, the timing of the exam does not establish the power of the clinician. Whereas long waits and short visits are the norm in many physicians' offices, in the alternative pelvic theater, the timing of scenes is reversed. Short waits and long visits are scheduled so that there is time for questions and explanations.

The issue of time reveals other less visible, but very important players in the traditional pelvic theater of operations: corporatized medicine with its chorus of inflated costs, unequal treatments, inaccessibility, drug industries, insurance companies, waste, and greed.[12] The economy of the alternative pelvic theater, its affordability and accessibility, is mandatory; otherwise, many are simply not allowed entrance into the theater in the first place.[13] While inevitably part of a capitalist system, the monetary ideals of alternative, woman-centered practice must revolve around self-sustenance rather than financial profit. Ironically, some ambitious marketers have recognized the increasing demand by "professional" women for woman-centered care. Clinics that market themselves as woman-

flaps and folds. I hope she doesn't think I'm strange. Linda assures me that everything looks healthy and normal. But it's an alien universe to me.

*

You decide you want to try inserting the speculum. You spread your vaginal lips and place the bills inside your vagina. You press the handles together and feel some pressure. You know when the pressure will start and how to make it stop. Your cervix is in view and you press the bottom handle down and into place. With a mirror in one hand and a flashlight in the other you illuminate your vagina. If you have a cervix, your reaction to first seeing it is:

(a) "Wow, I've never seen that before. It's really amazing."

(b) Wide eyes. Astonishment. Silence.

(c) "Oh my, I didn't know that was there."

(d) "Yuck, what's all that liquid. Is that OK?"

(e) Laughter.

(f) Uneasiness. Fear.

centered have sprung up throughout the country since the early 1980s. Their backers have redecorated the gynecological set with "womanly" attributes: soft lights, flowers, and pretty prints. But the costuming and roles of the pelvic theater remain indebted to conventional gynecological structures and access is limited to the paying few.[14] The traditional pelvic theater has simply received a new coat of soft pink paint.

The alternative theater of the speculative fiction incorporates the necessity of shifting roles. The collectively run clinic demands that all participants learn and perform a multiplicity of roles. There is no star performer who is beyond menial tasks. The health worker will perform practices usually executed by physicians, janitors, nurses, receptionists, and administrators. A collectively run clinic structurally disassembles the assembly-line method of standard care where, for example, the patient-product is passed from receptionist (who checks patient in, finds her chart) to nurse (who prepares patient for examination, may review history and even complete basic parts of the visit) to physician (who completes consult and examination) back to receptionist (who may then schedule appointments, receive payment, etc.).[15] The health worker who conducts almost every aspect of care confounds this traditional (and predominantly gendered) division of labor.[16] Also, the alternative pelvic theater encourages clinicians to

(g) "I won't have a hysterectomy for fibroids."

(h) To break into a serenade for your cervix.

(i) None of the above.

*

Jackie explains to me what a healthy cervix looks like, what the os is, the different types of secretions. There is this part of me—like an ear or a toe—that I never knew about. I've birthed and bled out of that tiny thing and I've never felt it, let alone seen it. I watch with the mirror as Jackie takes the pap smear sample. She describes each step of the process. I feel a numb rubbing sensation as she takes cells from different areas on, in, and around my cervix. Before I know it, we are done. It's strange. But I almost feel sad. I want to keep staring inside of me. I don't want to stop looking so soon. Jackie says I can remove the speculum and she'll wash it for me if I want to take it home. I accept. I feel like a child that just got a new Viewmaster. I am filled with excitement rather than dread. Why have I been so afraid of my own wetnesses and flesh? Was I simply afraid of the dark? Somehow, I don't think so.

Jackie explains the next part of the exam, the bimanual. She will insert two fingers into

work as a group, asking questions and conferring with each other when puzzled. Instead of dividing labor, the alternative pelvic theater distributes power differently from traditional gynecology.

Any practitioner, be she or he a physician, physician's assistant, nurse practitioner, or midwife, may adopt self-help practices and well-woman-related terminologies, and some have. But the more inculcated the practitioner is into a clinical system that situates the woman patient as passive, pathological, ignorant, and uneducable, the less likely the clinician will be to adopt alternative tools. The traditional gynecological apparatus is not equipped to accommodate such practices. Time and economic constraints may prohibit or discourage the clinician from seemingly time-consuming and "unnecessary" tasks like explaining the exam, helping the client to relax, or offering her a mirror.

In the alternative pelvic theater, the roles of clinician and client are not as fixed as in traditional gynecology; it is possible that the client may in turn train to become a health worker. In this speculative alternative, trainees are provided an education within clinic walls where they practice examination on each other and on other lay health workers. A rigorous training in well-woman gynecology would include alternative textbooks, readings, and lectures that do not pathologize female bodies and female performance. The woman-centered

my vagina, pressing on my abdomen with her other hand in order to check my ovaries and uterus. I've had this done many times before. I had this one doctor once who was very good at this. Very gentle. I didn't have insurance and later I found out he charged me $200. He didn't strike me as so wonderful after that. Jackie has a nice touch. Gentle and matter-of-fact.

*

I know I have fibroid tumors in my uterus. Linda says my uterus is about 10cm, about the size of a grapefruit, and asks what size it has been in the past. I wish I knew, but nobody ever told me. Four years ago a doctor found the fibroid tumors. She was poking around and said, "Well, you have tumors in your uterus. We'll monitor them. You may need a hysterectomy in the future." The words "tumor" and "hysterectomy" flipped out of her mouth as though they were second nature. Before I could ask anything, she left the room and came back with four medical students and started talking about me as though I wasn't there. "This is a thirty-year-old Hispanic female . . ." One by one without even asking me if I cared, she had the students stick fingers inside of me so they could feel my sick

pelvic apparatus must provide training, educational materials, and an environment that supports alternative practices and the individuals who perform them.

Touch

Stephen Tyler locates the "hegemony of the visual" in "Standard Average European thought and language." Other sensorial ways of knowing—tactility, smell, taste, sound—are continuously denigrated.[17] This notion of ocularcentrism is cohabitous with what Lakoff and Johnson label the "myths of objectivism and subjectivism," both of which "miss the way we *understand* the world through our *interactions* with it."[18] Western medicine's stake in objectivism, which Foucault historically links to the eighteenth century, is indeed ocularcentrically formulated. Because of the autopsy, pathology that was previously invisible became visible and therefore knowable. Western medicine is premised on the visible—seeing is believing and knowing.

In Western medicine, there is often a distrust of touch. The physician sometimes uses fingers/palpation/touch as an initial tool, a scout, but if touch detects a problem, a visual assessment is required to confirm and define—a biopsy, an

insides. And a *woman* doctor was putting me through all of this. I was stunned. But the thought of cancer overrode my shock and dread of being examined by four students. Cancer, I thought. Cancer. Cancer. The doctor and students disappeared without a word. I went home, prepared my things, wrote up a will. My lover couldn't handle the stress. Our relationship ended. But the doctor hadn't told me how long I had. For three months I was afraid to ask. I finally called her up and she seemed very humored by my ignorance. She patronized me. "Fibroid tumors are benign, NONcancerous. You don't have cancer."

Linda asks me if I want to feel my own uterus. This is a frightening idea, but I want to know what those students felt that day. I nod and she puts my hand on my lower belly while she lifts up my cervix with her inside hand. Sure enough. There it is. Incredible. She says that fibroids are very common and that she'd like one of the doctors to come in and repeat the exam in order to monitor the fibroids. Linda leaves the room and brings back the doctor. She introduces herself as Maria and is just as nice as Linda. Very gentle and explains what she is doing. She tells me that fibroids are probably what cause me pain and clotting with my periods. She says many women have had good luck with Chinese herbs.

ultrasound (where sound becomes visible), an X ray. In certain non-Western practices, such as traditional Chinese medicine, the quality of a felt pulse—its "slipperiness," its "deepness"—may tell more about the condition of the whole body than any visual proof. But the *ocular* vocabulary of Western medicine is more elaborate than any tactile vocabulary. Given this, how can we discuss the quality of the clinician's contact with the patient's body?

Within the pelvic exam, the clinician's quality of touch and the woman patient's experience of such contact is critical in considering the quality of the exam. In chapter 4, I explored the ways images of female genitals, regardless of their intended audience, can be read as clinical or sexual or both. Likewise, when a woman's genital's are touched she may "read" the quality of that touch as clinical or sexual or as some combination of the two, despite the intentions of the clinician. This is partly due to the fact that for some women, particularly sexual abuse survivors, genital manipulation has been linked with emotional trauma, fear, and vulnerability. Such abuse has often taken place in an instance where a woman or girl feels she has no control. A pelvic exam in which a woman or girl feels she has no control may also replicate the initial situation's horror for her.

Many times, the seemingly uninvasive act of having her genitals *observed* by a clinician, the unveiling or lifting of the drape, causes a woman severe anxiety.

Their fibroids have decreased in size dramatically. Though sometimes women prefer surgery. She can give me a referral for an herbalist. I'll take it.

*

These women came to this park near my house and parked their van there. Actually, it was more like an RV with a ramp. They called it a Mobile Pap Unit. Fancy name, and it was pretty cool on the inside. It had these little rooms, each one had a pap table in it, electric so people in wheelchairs could get in and out. They said I should pay what I could. They spoke a bunch of different languages. Some of them were outside passing out information about health stuff and just talking to people. It's hard for me to get out much. But they came to my park so I didn't have to leave the neighborhood. I never had a pap before.

*

Doris, my lover, and I have been thinking about having a baby. She wants to get pregnant, but we don't have any male friend who we can really ask to help us with sperm. Linda says the center has an alternative insemination program for lesbians and single straight women. Ask and ye shall receive. Not quite that easy; frozen sperm is expensive and the demand for

Michael Taussig's discussion of the implicit relationship between the visual and tactile offers one way of understanding this horror: "elementary physics and physiology might instruct that these two features of copy and contact are steps in the same process, that a ray of light, for example, moves from the rising sun into the human eye where it makes *contact* with the retinal rods and cones to form, via the circuits of the central nervous system, a (culturally attuned) *copy* of the rising sun. On this line of reasoning, contact and copy merge to become virtually identical, different moments of the one process of sensing; seeing something or hearing something is to be in contact with that something."[19] In effect, Taussig reframes the visual act, the act of looking, as a tactile act, an act of touching. Therefore, there is an "unstoppable merging of the object of perception with the body of the perceiver and not just with the mind's eye."[20] To apply Taussig's statements to the pelvic exam, "the object of perception" or the woman patient's genitals are merging with "the body of the perceiver" or the clinician's body. In an attempt to theoretically dismantle the primacy of the visual and its attending "myth of objectivism," Taussig's notion of the relationship between the tactile and the visual (and aural) implicates the viewer in making contact or interacting with the object of the gaze. There can be no such thing as a distanced observer.

Taussig's interpretation may also be helpful in considering the importance of

this service is great. Linda says one of the reasons the waiting list is so long is because many other insemination programs demand that women who are unmarried—lesbian or straight—undergo a battery of psychological tests to prove they will be fit parents. Unreal.

*

Gathering my pap smear packet and my speculum, Jackie says I can get dressed on the bottom and undressed on top so we can do a breast exam and leaves the room. I've always felt like a cow during a breast exam. Squeezed and prodded and I'm expected to stare at the ceiling and chew cud or something. Hey, lighten up, I always wanted to say, these may be fatty, cancer-producing sacks to you, but they mean a lot more to me. But I didn't. I just chewed and chewed.

I sit on the table, naked from the waist up. Jackie enters and does not hold a conversation with my boobs, but looks at my eyes. We discuss breast self-exam. I instantly feel guilty. "I know. I know I should do it." But Jackie has a way of encouraging me and telling me how important it is to examine my breasts without making me feel bad. One of the reasons I don't do it is that I don't really know what I'm looking for. It all feels like lumps

"eye contact," more specifically the *intermittent* act of the clinician seeking out the client's gaze, within the gynecological exam. If being viewed and touched is synonymous with a kind of powerless horror that renders the clinician an active pursuer and the client a passive receptor, eye contact may allow the patient to play a more active role in the exam. Although the patient is being looked at and touched, if she has the potential to return the clinician's gaze she is able to participate in a kind of "looking back" and "touching back" that could alter her feelings of powerlessness. It is indeed possible that a client could be uncomfortable with such eye contact and therefore avoid the clinician's gaze by averting her eyes. However, by attempting to make eye contact, the clinician has given the client an option.

Discussions of self-touch for the purpose of self-pleasure can be incorporated into alternative self-help practice. In mainstream practice, female sexuality is largely disavowed within the context of the exam. While a woman's sexual history is discussed, issues surrounding pleasure or pain with touch are ignored or, due to the structure of the exam, never surface in the first place. Discussions about and information regarding orgasm, masturbation, and other sexual pleasures must not be disavowed within the alternative, woman-centered pelvic theater. Ideally, the flexibility of the alternative theater and the degree of comfort produced within that scenario enables the client to learn more about her own

to me, plus I'm terrified of finding something. Jackie assures me about the good outcomes of early cancer detection and then takes me through all the steps, explaining exactly what I'm looking for in the mirror—dimpling, puckering, lumps—and then what I'm feeling for. She tells me that most women have breasts with a lumpy texture and gives me good tricks for imagining what I'm feeling for: "a pea in lumpy mashed potatoes" or "a marble under a rug." She has me feel normal lumpy breast texture so I don't confuse that with other lumps. We talk about mammograms and all the pros and cons. She knows about all these different studies. She gives me information so I can decide for myself. She gives me the most thorough exam I've ever had, really checking each inch of my breast. Before, I've had doctors tell me how important it is to do thorough self-breast-exam while they're breezing across my breasts like they're hot potatoes. That makes you wonder whether you're supposed to do like they say or like they do. We're done and I silently promise myself to try to check my breasts more often now that I really know how. Jackie leaves. I get dressed, meeting her back at our table and chairs. She hands me my speculum. It is a trophy, I think, as I put it in my bag.

sexuality and sexual pleasures, including masturbation and orgasm. No longer is the woman positioned as passive, desexualized object, but rather she is encouraged to voice questions about her own desires and pleasures.[21]

Speculation

What is speculative is *theoretical, not demonstrable.* The speculative fiction is theoretical, not demonstrable, a narrative composite of history, theory, anecdote, and speculation—a conscious blend of true and false that supports a consideration of alternative, woman-centered practice.

Speculative fiction is science fiction. In this case, speculative fiction = science fiction + speculums.

The practice of gynecology itself is speculation. Built into its very structure is a dependence on spectatorship and the speculum. But the performance of gynecology also incorporates the notion of speculation in terms of speculating the future, a speculation indebted to past and present performances. In the many performances of gynecology new futures are imagined. Each choice made as to how exams are practiced and represented situates women—their agency, sexualities, and bodies.

Representations and practices form what is the "heterogenous ensemble" that constitutes the gynecological apparatus. These chapters have located a select cast from this ensemble—a cast of various publics and privates. Each chapter explores a particular node of pelvic exam performance. The divisions between these chapters are not absolute. The performance of each leaves its trace on the others. In an infinite number of combinations, each member of the ensemble interacts with the other members, whether in collusion, through critique, or in some complicated relationship beyond such clear-cut possibilities. Within each chapter can be found suggestions for how each part of the ensemble relates to the larger apparatus. The gynecological apparatus is as much defined by what lies within each chapter as by what occurs in the interstices. In these spaces, suggested within and between the chapters, one can see how the twins' creation of the Mantle retractor in *Dead Ringers* may be indebted to Sims's "discovery" of the speculum and may in turn inspire new frontiers and fears of gynecological innovation. One may find that Annie Sprinkle's "Public Cervix Announcement" is a loud, reprimanding scream at gynecological textbook images that position women's genitals as clinical, as well as a taunt at medical educators to reconsider their use of prostitutes as pelvic models. One can find that a consideration of self-spectatorship, specifically cervical self-exam, within woman-centered practice is a plea to reconsider the nurse hired as the first pelvic model, draped so her face was covered in order to remain anonymous. The interconnections are numerous and productive.

These speculations are an "investment" in some intended outcome. At the base of these critical writings is a concern with changing the gynecological apparatus. But this change is not a matter of simply plugging a new variable into the apparatus—either women physicians or gynecology teaching associates or homey, soft pink exam rooms. To overhaul the apparatus is to introduce entirely different structures and models.[22] The positions of spectator-spectacle, director-actress, and clinician-patient must be denaturalized and questioned. Rather, consider the possibility of theater (pelvic or otherwise) without a director. Instead of obeying a single vision, consider the multiple perspectives that could be brought to such a practice. What I am calling for is a change in how we conceptualize and create new practices and representations combined with a recognition that practices and representations are interdependent and, at times, even one and the same.

Gynecology is not a sealed entity. It is leaky. Its practices and representations are indebted to and productive of greater cultural attitudes about female bodies and sexualities. I have no desire to police the boundaries that lie so precariously between gynecology and other cultural forms. Rather I wish to recognize the fluidity across boundaries and to use that discovery in order to encourage and support the creation of new performances.

Notes

Introduction: Public Privates

1   Mary Russo, "Female Grotesques: Carnival and Theory," in *Feminist Studies/Critical Studies*, ed. Teresa de Lauretis (Bloomington: Indiana University Press, 1986), p. 213.

2   Michel Foucault, *The Birth of the Clinic: An Archaeology of Medical Perception*, trans. A. M. Sheridan Smith (New York: Random House, 1973).

3   On the false binary "between the power of visibility and the impotency of invisibility," see Peggy Phelan, *Unmarked: the Politics of Performance* (New York: Routledge, 1993), p. 6.

1   The Performance of Pelvics

1   James M. Henslin and Mae A. Biggs, "Dramaturgical Desexualization: The Sociology of Vaginal Examination," in *Studies in the Sociology of Sex*, ed. James M. Henslin (New York: Appleton-Century-Crofts, 1971), p. 244.

2   Ibid., pp. 251–52.

3   Ibid., p. 258, original emphasis.

4   Ibid., p. 265.

5   Ibid., pp. 266–67.

6   Judith Butler, *Bodies That Matter* (New York: Routledge, 1993), p. 237.

7   While teaching pelvic exams, I heard about various educators who instruct their clothed male students to assume the lithotomy position on gynecological exam tables so that they might begin to understand how such a posture positions their patients.

8   Elaine Showalter, *The Female Malady: Women, Madness, and English Culture, 1830–1980* (New York: Viking Penguin, 1985), p. 148.

9   Bernard R. Shochet, M.D., Leon A. Levin, M.D., and Ephraim T. Lisansky, M.D., "Roundtable: The Seductive Patient," *Medical Aspects of Human Sexuality* 16, no. 1 (January 1982): 36K.

10 Ibid., p. 36L.

11 Joan P. Emerson, "Behavior in Private Places: Sustaining Definitions of Reality in Gynecological Examinations," in *Recent Sociology No. 2: Patterns of Communicative Behavior*, ed. Hans Peter Dreitzel (London: Macmillan, 1970), p. 87.

12 Henslin and Biggs, "Dramaturgical Desexualization," p. 271 n. 15.

13 Ibid., p. 272.

14 Mary Douglas, *Purity and Danger: An Analysis of Concepts of Pollution and Taboo* (London: Routledge, 1966).

15 Lynda Nead, *The Female Nude: Art, Obscenity and Sexuality* (London: Routledge, 1992), p. 6.

16 On the grotesque body, see Mikhail Bakhtin, *Rabelais and His World*, trans. Helene Iswolsky (Bloomington: Indiana University Press, 1984). Also see Peter Stalleybrass and Allon White, *The Politics and Poetics of Transgression* (Ithaca: Cornell University Press, 1986). For a brilliant consideration of the female grotesque, see Russo, "Female Grotesques."

17 Christian Metz, "The Imaginary Signifier [Excerpts]," in *Narrative, Apparatus, Ideology*, ed. Philip Rosen (New York: Columbia University Press, 1986), pp. 263–64.

18 Emily Martin, *The Woman in the Body: A Cultural Analysis of Reproduction* (Boston: Beacon Press, 1987), p. 74.

19 Jill Dolan, *Presence and Desire* (Ann Arbor: University of Michigan Press, 1993).

20 Ludmilla Jordanova, *Sexual Visions: Images of Gender in Science and Medicine between the Eighteenth and Twentieth Centuries* (Madison: University of Wisconsin Press, 1989).

21 Giuliana Bruno, "Spectatorial Embodiments: Anatomies of the Visible and the Female Bodyscape," *Camera Obscura* 28 (January 1992): 241.

22 Ibid., p. 243.

23 Laura Mulvey, "Visual Pleasure and Narrative Cinema," *Screen* 16, no. 3 (autumn 1975): 6–18.

24 John M. Smith, M.D., *Women and Doctors* (New York: Atlantic Monthly Press, 1992), p. 115.

25 Ibid., p. 32.

26 Sue V. Rosser makes a similar proposal: place more women in decision-making positions in such areas as clinical research and the medical institution will change. See *Women's Health: Missing from U.S. Medicine* (Bloomington: University of Indiana Press, 1994), pp. 10–13.

27 A proliferation of texts considering the female spectator followed Mulvey's "Visual Pleasure and Narrative Cinema": Janet Bergstrom and Mary Ann Doane, eds., *Camera Obscura* 20–21 (May–September 1989); E. Deidre Pribram, ed., *Female Spectators: Looking at Film and Television* (London: Verso, 1988); Lorraine Gamman and Margaret Marshment, eds., *The Female Gaze: Women as Viewers of Popular Culture* (Seattle: Real Comet Press, 1989).

28 Laura Mulvey, "Afterthoughts on 'Visual Pleasure and Narrative Cinema' inspired by King Vidor's *Duel in the Sun* (1946)," in *Visual and Other Pleasures* (Bloomington: Indiana University Press, 1989), p. 31.

29 Mary Ann Doane, *The Desire to Desire* (Bloomington: Indiana University Press, 1987), p. 67.

30 Laura Kipnis, *Ecstasy Unlimited: On Sex, Capital, Gender, and Aesthetics* (Minneapolis: University of Minnesota Press, 1993), pp. 8–9.

31 For example, Thomas A. King, "Performing 'Akimbo': Queer Pride and Epistemological Prejudice," in *Politics and Poetics of Camp*, ed. Moe Meyer (New York: Routledge, 1994), pp. 23–50;

Kate Davy, "Fe-Male Impersonation: The Discourse of Camp," in *Politics and Poetics of Camp*, pp. 130–48; Alexander Doty, *Making Things Perfectly Queer: Interpreting Mass Culture* (Minneapolis: University of Minnesota Press, 1993); Richard Dyer, ed., *Gays in Film* (London: BFI, 1980); Judith Mayne, "The Critical Audience," in *Cinema and Spectatorship* (New York: Routledge, 1993), pp. 157–72.

32 It is clear that heterosexism will actually affect whether women seek care. Susan Gilbert, "Bias in Doctors' Offices May Harm Gay Women's Health, Study Finds," *New York Times*, October 11, 1995.

33 Peggy Phelan, *Unmarked: The Politics of Performance* (New York: Routledge, 1993), p. 4.

34 Elin Diamond, "Brechtian Theory/Feminist Theory: Toward a Gestic Feminist Criticism," *Drama Review* 32, no. 1 (1988): 90.

35 Ibid., p. 83.

36 Jean-Louis Baudry, "Ideological Effects of the Basic Cinematographic Apparatus," *Narrative, Apparatus, Ideology*, ed. Philip Rosen (New York: Columbia University Press, 1988), p. 288.

37 Philip Rosen, introduction to Part 3 in *Narrative, Apparatus, Ideology*, p. 282.

38 The pelvic exam apparatus, like the cinematic apparatus, is what Teresa de Lauretis refers to as a "technology of gender." See *Technologies of Gender* (Bloomington: Indiana University Press, 1987), p. 13.

39 Michel Foucault, *Power/Knowledge: Selected Interviews and Other Writings 1972–1977*, ed. Colin Gordon (New York: Pantheon, 1972), pp. 194–96.

40 See Michel deCerteau, *Practice of Everyday Life*, trans. Steven Rendall (Berkeley: University of California Press, 1984), pp. xi–xxiv.

41 Phelan, *Unmarked*, p. 3.

42 See Linda Montano, *Art in Everyday Life* (New York: Station Hill, 1981). See also Andrea Juno and V. Vale, eds., "Linda Montano," in *Angry Women* (San Francisco: Re/Search Publications, 1991), pp. 50–65.

43 Phelan, *Unmarked*, p. 148.

44 Ibid., pp. 148–49.

45 In describing the work of Angelika Festa, for instance, Phelan does not discuss the fact that her performances are multimedia, incorporating multiple mass-reproduced technologies (see Phelan, *Unmarked*, pp. 152–58). For an example of how a nonmechanically technological performance can still be indebted to mass reproduction, see Margaret Thompson Drewal, "From Rocky's Rockettes to Liberace: The Politics of Representation in the Heart of Corporate Capitalism," *Journal of American Culture* 10, no. 2 (summer 1987): 69–82.

2 Mastering the Female Pelvis

1 J. Chassar Moir, *The Vesico-Vaginal Fistula*, 2d ed. (London: Bailliere Tindall and Cassell, 1967), p. 16. This epigraph is an excerpt from the introductory chapter, "J. Marion Sims and the Vesico-vaginal Fistula: Then and Now," which was originally an address given to the Oxford University Medical Society, October 1940.

2 See Jessica Mitford, *The American Way of Birth* (New York: Dutton, 1992), p. 39. Mitford's discussion of Sims is largely based on G. J. Barker-Benfield, *The Horrors of the Half-Known Life* (New York: Harper & Row, 1976), ch. 10: "Architect of the Vagina."

3 Mitford, *American Way of Birth*, 39. Irwin H. Kaiser, M.D., states that "Sims and the other

gynecological surgeons made their money by applying the hospital discoveries [made on slaves and poor white women] in private practice, where they charged stupendous fees." See his article, "Reappraisals of J. Marion Sims," *American Journal of Obstetrics and Gynecology* 132 (1978): 878.

4   Seale Harris, M.D., *Woman's Surgeon: The Life Story of J. Marion Sims* (New York: Macmillan, 1950), p. 107.

5   Historically, there has been a connection between circus freaks and medical institutions. In London, for example, physicians were sought after to bless new freak shows with reviews declaring the verity of their freakishness. Often medical men would denounce the show, but then later they would purchase the skeletons of dead freaks in order to display them at the medical school. See Richard Daniel Altick, *The Shows of London* (Cambridge, Mass.: Harvard University Press, 1978), p. 260.

6   A. H. Saxon, *P. T. Barnum: The Legend and the Man* (New York: Columbia University Press, 1989), p. 79.

7   Ibid., pp. 76, 99.

8   Ibid., p. 68.

9   Ibid., p. 71.

10 J. Marion Sims, M.D., *The Story of My Life*, ed. H. Marion-Sims, M.D. (New York: D. Appleton and Company, 1886), p. 231.

11 Moir, *Vesico-Vaginal Fistula*, p. 2.

12 Elizabeth Fox-Genovese, *Within the Plantation Household: Black and White Women of the South* (Chapel Hill: University of North Carolina Press, 1988), p. 171. Also see Deborah Gray White, *Ar'n't I a Woman?: Female Slaves in the Plantation South* (New York: W. W. Norton, 1985), pp. 124–25.

13 W. O. Baldwin, "Tribute to the Late James Marion Sims, November, 1883," in *The Story of My Life*, by J. Marion Sims, p. 429.

14 Harris, *Woman's Surgeon*, p. 95.

15 Sims, *Story of My Life*, p. 23.

16 Ibid., p. 277.

17 John D'Emilio and Estelle B. Freedman, *Intimate Matters: A History of Sexuality in America* (New York: Harper & Row, 1988), pp. 99–100. D'Emilio and Freedman cite Angela Davis's discussion of the value slave women placed on motherhood for their own reasons. See Angela Davis, "The Black Woman's Role in the Community of Slaves," *Black Scholar* 3 (December 1971): 2.

18 White, *Ar'n't I a Woman?* pp. 79–80.

19 D'Emilio and Freedman, *Intimate Matters*, p. 94.

20 While an undeniably unpleasant condition for women to have, it is important to note that fistulas usually do not affect a woman's ability to conceive.

21 White, *Ar'n't I a Woman?* p. 80. Todd L. Savitt, "Black Health on the Plantation: Masters, Slaves, and Physicians," in *Science and Medicine in the Old South*, ed. Ronald L. Numbers and Todd L. Savitt (Baton Rouge: Louisiana State University Press, 1989), p. 345.

22 White, *Ar'n't I a Woman?* p. 82.

23 Sims, *Story of My Life*, p. 230.

24 Many of the normal positions of the uterus were considered pathological in the early practice of gynecology; thus "replacing the uterus" was a common procedure. For example, in Henry T. Byford's *Manual of Gynecology* (Philadelphia: P. Blakiston, 1897), there is a description of the maneuver that Sims learned as a medical student: "The uterus may be replaced by putting the

patient in the knee-chest position (Campbell), admitting air to the vagina, and pushing the fundus toward the promontory of the sacrum with a blunt instrument like a drumstick. . . . When the fundus is dislodged from the hollow of the sacrum, gravity completes the replacement. This is a good method for the replacement of the pregnant uterus" (p. 246). A number of physical and mental disorders were linked to the uterus. "Local treatments" to the uterus consisting of manual relocation, leeches, and "injections" of various substances were common practice. See Ann Douglas Wood, " 'The Fashionable Diseases': Women's Complaints and Their Treatment in Nineteenth-Century America," in *Women and Health in America*, ed. Judith Walzer Leavitt (Madison: University of Wisconsin Press, 1984), pp. 222–38.

25 Sims, *Story of My Life*, pp. 234–35.

26 See Harold Speert, M.D., *Obstetric and Gynecologic Milestones* (New York: Macmillan, 1958), pp. 447–49.

27 Baldwin, "Tribute," p. 434.

28 See Mary Ann Doane, "Dark Continents: Epistemologies of Racial and Sexual Difference in Psychoanalysis and the Cinema," in *Femmes Fatales: Feminism, Film Theory, Psychoanalysis* (New York: Routledge, 1991), pp. 209–48.

29 Mary Ann Doane, *The Desire to Desire* (Bloomington: Indiana University Press, 1987), p. 61.

30 See Michel Foucault, *The Birth of the Clinic: An Archaeology of Medical Perception*, trans. A. M. Sheridan Smith (New York: Random House, 1973).

31 Baldwin, "Tribute," p. 434.

32 Sims, *Story of My Life*, p. 235.

33 Donna Haraway locates this trope of the "hero-scientist" in an immunology textbook from 1987. She maintains that "science remains an important genre of Western exploration and travel literature." See Haraway, "The Biopolitics of Postmodern Bodies: Constitutions of Self in Immune System Discourse," in *Simians, Cyborgs, and Women: The Reinvention of Nature* (New York: Routledge, 1991), p. 205.

34 Teresa de Lauretis, *Alice Doesn't: Feminism, Semiotics, Cinema* (Bloomington: Indiana University Press, 1984), pp. 127–28.

35 Sims, *Story of My Life*, p. 236.

36 Ibid., p. 237.

37 Harris, *Woman's Surgeon*, p. 99.

38 Diana E. Axelsen, "Women as Victims of Medical Experimentation: J. Marion Sims' Surgery on Slave Women, 1845–50," *Sage* 2, no. 2 (fall 1985): 11. Axelsen questions "Sims' continued failure to use ether or to seek out current research in the area of anesthesiology." She implies that no attempt was made on Sims's part to help alleviate the slave women's pain.

39 Sander L. Gilman, "Black Bodies, White Bodies: Toward an Iconography of Female Sexuality in Late Nineteenth-Century Art, Medicine, and Literature," *Critical Inquiry* (autumn 1985): 231. Winthrop D. Jordan, *White over Black: American Attitudes toward the Negro, 1550–1812* (New York: W. W. Norton, 1968), pp. 517–21.

40 Black *male* sexuality was undeniably constructed as pathological too. But the link between black female sexuality and genitalia was repeatedly drawn, whereas black male genitalia were left out of the discussion. When Gilman examines autopsy reports from the late nineteenth century, he finds that black female genitalia are discussed but that there is no discussion of black male genitalia whatsoever. See Gilman, "Black Bodies, White Bodies," p. 218.

41 For a discussion of this dichotomy, see Hazel Carby, "Slave and Mistress: Ideologies of Womanhood under Slavery," in *Reconstructing Womanhood: The Emergence of the Afro-American Woman Novelist* (New York: Oxford University Press, 1987), pp. 20–39.

42 Sander L. Gilman, *Difference and Pathology: Stereotypes of Sex, Race, and Madness* (Ithaca: Cornell University Press, 1985), p. 88.

43 Ibid., p. 88 n. 19. For a contemporary take on the Hottentot Venus, see Lisa Jones, "Venus Envy," in *Bulletproof Diva: Tales of Race, Sex, and Hair* (New York: Anchor Books, 1994), pp. 73–77.

44 Ludmilla Jordanova, *Sexual Visions: Images of Gender in Science and Medicine between the Eighteenth and Twentieth Centuries* (Madison: University of Wisconsin Press, 1989), pp. 138–39.

45 See Harris, *Woman's Surgeon*, p. 98. Historically, Africans and in turn African slaves were considered to be beasts, thus making them particularly fitting "guinea pigs." See Jordan, *White over Black*, pp. 228–34. See also Todd L. Savitt, "The Use of Blacks for Medical Experimentation and Demonstration in the Old South," *Journal of Southern History* 48, no. 3 (August 1982): 332.

46 Sims, *Story of My Life*, p. 470.

47 Axelsen, "Women as Victims," p. 12.

48 Sims, *Story of My Life*, p. 241.

49 Ibid.

50 This is not to belittle the great achievements of black female health care professionals regardless of their role, but rather to point to the fact that black women have often been excluded from positions of power within the medical establishment. Black women have had to fight tremendously hard for inclusion even as assistants. See Darlene Clark Hine, "Mabel K. Stauper and the Integration of Black Nurses into the Armed Forces," in *Women and Health in America*, ed. Judith Walzer Leavitt (Madison: University of Wisconsin Press, 1984), pp. 497–506. For exceptions to the idea of limited roles for black women in the health professions, see Sheila P. Davis and Cora A. Ingram, "Empowered Caretakers: A Historical Perspective on the Roles of Granny Midwives in Rural Alabama," in *Wings of Gauze: Women of Color and the Experience of Health and Illness*, ed. Barbara Bair and Susan E. Cayleff (Detroit: Wayne State University Press, 1993), pp. 191–201; and Melissa Blount, "Surpassing Obstacles: Pioneering Black Women Physicians," in *The Black Women's Health Book: Speaking for Ourselves*, ed. Evelyn C. White (Seattle: Seal Press, 1990), pp. 44–51.

51 Harris, *Woman's Surgeon*, p. 99.

52 Durrenda Ojanuga, "The Medical Ethics of the 'Father of Gynaecology,' Dr. J. Marion Sims," *Journal of Medical Ethics* 19 (1993): 28–31. See also Todd L. Savitt, *Medicine and Slavery: The Diseases and Health Care of Blacks in Ante-bellum Virginia* (Urbana: University of Illinois Press, 1978), p. 293.

53 Harris, *Woman's Surgeon*, p. 92.

54 Cited in Barker-Benfield, *Horrors of the Half-Known Life*, p. 96.

55 Barbara Ehrenreich and Deirdre English, *For Her Own Good: 150 Years of the Experts' Advice to Women* (New York: Doubleday, 1978), p. 125.

56 Harris, *Woman's Surgeon*, p. 109.

57 Barker-Benfield, *Horrors of the Half-Known Life* , pp. 102–3.

58 Ibid., p. 98.

59 Sims, *Story of My Life*, p. 295.

60 See Lawrence D. Longo, "The Rise and Fall of Battey's Operation: A Fashion in Surgery," in *Women and Health in America*, ed. Judith Walzer Leavitt (Madison: University of Wisconsin Press, 1984), p. 270.

61 See Harris, *Woman's Surgeon*, p. 298.

62 Ibid., pp. 129, 135, 288.

63 See Barker-Benfield, *Horrors of the Half-Known Life*, p. 110.

64 Ibid, p. 105.

65 Kaiser, "Reappraisals of J. Marion Sims," p. 878. See also S. Buford Word, M.D., "The Father of Gynecology," *Alabama Journal of Medical Science* 9, no. 1 (1972): 33–39.

66 The front cover of Wyeth-Ayerst Laboratories' Norplant information booklet for consumers reads: "Would you like up to 5 years of continuous birth control that is reversible? Welcome to a new era in contraceptive technology."

67 I find one volume on Norplant particularly helpful. See Barbara Mintzes, Anita Hardon, and Jannemieke Hanhart, eds., *Norplant: Under Her Skin* (Amsterdam: Women's Health Action Foundation, 1993), p. 90.

68 White, *Ar'n't I a Woman?* p. 98.

69 Robert Pear, "Population Growth Outstrips Earlier U.S. Census Estimates," *New York Times*, December 4, 1992.

70 Tamar Lewin, "Baltimore School Clinics to Offer Birth Control by Surgical Implant," *New York Times*, December 4, 1992.

71 Thomas M. Shapiro, *Population Control Politics: Women, Sterilization, and Reproductive Choice* (Philadelphia: Temple University Press, 1985), p. 118. This very term was used during slavery to refer to slave women who could reproduce efficiently. See White, *Ar'n't I a Woman?* p. 105.

72 See Faye Wattleton, "Using Birth Control as Coercion," *Los Angeles Times*, January 13, 1991.

73 See Stacey L. Arthur, "The Norplant Prescription: Birth Control, Woman Control, or Crime Control?" *UCLA Law Review* 40, no. 1 (1992): 1–101; and Gretchen Long, "Norplant: A Victory, Not a Panacea for Poverty," *National Lawyers Guild Practitioner* 50, no. 1 (winter 1993): 11–13. The attempt to control African American reproduction by means of the judicial system has a long and sordid history. See Dorothy E. Roberts, "Crime, Race, and Reproduction," *Tulane Law Review* 67 (1993): 1945–77.

74 Shana Morrow, "Welfare Reform and Reproductive Freedom," Planned Parenthood, Chicago Area, "Political Affairs Perspective" (fall 1993): 2–3, 7.

75 National Black Women's Health Project, "Facts: Norplant" (newsletter) 1992.

76 Issues of "choice" and informed consent haunt another set of medical experiments that occurred about eighty years following Sims's experiments and less than forty miles from Montgomery. These experiments, which happened in and around Tuskegee county, were nontherapeutic, meaning no new technology (e.g., surgery or device) was being tried. This time poor, illiterate African American men were the subjects, not slave women. Men were chosen who had been infected with syphilis, but who were never told that they had syphilis. Instead the white Public Health Service (PHS) practitioners told them they had "bad blood." In exchange for being part of the study, the men received free physical exams, lunch on the day of the exam, and burial insurance. No treatment was ever given; instead their slow physical and/or psychological deterioration was monitored over the course of forty years (1932–72). This study has been superbly documented by James H. Jones in his book *Bad Blood: The Tuskegee Syphilis Experiment.*

 At first sight, it might seem as though Sims's work and the PHS study have little in common other than geographical proximity. Yet both projects are founded on similar attitudes regarding black bodies, black sexuality, and the relationship of these bodies and sexualities to pathology. Both syphilis and vesico-vaginal fistulas are conditions related to genitalia and therefore sexuality. Syphilis is a sexually transmitted disease that is often associated with sexual promiscuity. The contraction and transmission of the disease was therefore readily associated with African Americans. As Jones notes, "No disease seemed more suited to blacks than syphilis, for physicians were certain that exaggerated libido and sexual promiscuity had led to a high incidence of the disease among blacks." Both Sims's and the PHS's experiments are symptomatic of a pathological, white-dominated medical mindset that devalues black bodies. Why not let these societally less powerful people experience prolonged suffering and pain? Suffering and pain might lead either to reparation or to death depending on the desires of those officiating the "treatments." The slave woman would be more helpful repaired; the poor black man after slavery would be more useful dead.

77 Robert A. Hatcher, M.D., M.P.H. et al., *Contraceptive Technology 1990–1992*, 15th rev. ed. (New York: Irvington, 1994), p. 307.

78 Mintzes, Hardon, and Hanhart, *Norplant*, p. 10.

79 The Population Council, "Norplant Worldwide" no. 16 (November 1991): 2.

80 American Health Consultants, "Clinicians, Patients, Medicaid: Is Anyone to Blame for Norplant Removal Dilemma?" *Contraceptive Technology Update* 14, no. 10 (October 1993): 152.

81 Native American Women's Health Education Resource Center, *The Impact of Norplant in the Native American Community* (June 1992): 13.

82 The back cover of Wyeth-Ayerst Laboratories' Norplant information booklet for consumers reads: "Ask your doctor if the Norplant System is right for you . . . It's your choice."

83 Mintzes, Hardon, and Hanhart, *Norplant*, p. 90.

84 Betsey Hartmann, *Reproductive Rights and Wrongs: The Global Politics of Population Control and Contraceptive Choice* (New York: Harper & Row, 1987), p. 232.

85 Ibid.

86 Ibid., p. 213.

87 Ibid., p. 241.

88 See Shapiro, *Population Control*, p. 107.

89 Cited in Hartmann, *Reproductive Rights*, p. 241.

90 Eeva Ollila, Kristiina Kajesalo, and Elina Hemminki, "Experience of Norplant by Finnish Family Planning Practitioners," in *Norplant: Under Her Skin*, ed. Mintzes, Hardon, and Hanhart, p. 61.

91 Ibid. Here the authors cite A. Purvis, "A Pill That Gets under the Skin: Norplant Could Spur Birth Control—and Stir Controversy," *Time* (December 24, 1990): 45.

92 Hartmann, *Reproductive Rights*, p. 200.

93 *Jane Doe, Annrita Garcia, Mary Roe, and Leticia Walker* v *Wyeth-Ayerst Laboratories*, 93 L 11096. See Heather M. Little, "No Panacea: Norplant Suit Charges Failure to Educate Patients," *Chicago Tribune*, October 31, 1993.

94 Inadequate counseling and informed consent as well as the practice of inserting Norplant in women who are medically at risk has been well documented within the Native American community. See Native American Women's Health Education Resource Center, *Impact of Norplant*. An overview of this study was printed as "Native American Women Uncover Norplant Abuses," *Ms.* (September/October 1993): 69.

95 See American Health Consultants, "Too Much or Too Little—Access to Norplant Implants Fuels Ethics Debate," *Contraceptive Technology Update* 14, no. 9 (September 1993); and "Clinicians, Patients, Medicaid: Is Anyone to Blame for Norplant Removal Dilemma?" *Contraceptive Technology Update* 14, no. 10 (October 1993).

96 Barker-Benfield, *Horrors of the Half-Known Life*, p. 95.

3   Cadavers, Dolls, and Prostitutes

1 Quoted in Robert M. Kretzschmar, M.D., "Evolution of the Gynecology Teaching Associate: An Education Specialist," *American Journal of Obstetrics and Gynecology* 131, no. 4 (June 15, 1978): 373; italics added.

2 Julius Buchwald, M.D., "The First Pelvic Examination: Helping Students Cope with Their Emotional Reactions," *Journal of Medical Education* 54 (September 1979): 725–28.

3 A. M. Sheridan Smith, translator's note to *The Birth of the Clinic: An Archaeology of Medical Perception*, by Michel Foucault (New York: Random House, 1973), p. vii.

4 See Louis Vontver, M.D., et al., "The Effects of Two Methods of Pelvic Examination Instruction on Student Performance and Anxiety," *Journal of Medical Education* 55 (September 1980): 778–85. Here elaborate methods are used to monitor student stress—researchers employed EKGS—whereas little consideration is paid to patient's comfort. Shouldn't EKGS have been used to monitor the patients' stress levels?

5 Buchwald, "First Pelvic Examination," p. 726.

6 Laura Mulvey, "Afterthoughts on 'Visual Pleasure and Narrative Cinema' inspired by King Vidor's *Duel in the Sun* (1946)," in *Visual and Other Pleasures* (Bloomington: Indiana University Press, 1989), p. 33.

7 I did find mention of the use of anesthetized women in teaching students how to do pelvic exams. See Ralph W. Hale, M.D., and Wilma Schiner, R. N., "Professional Patients: An Improved Method of Teaching Breast and Pelvic Examination," *Journal of Reproductive Medicine* 19, no. 3 (September 1977): 163; Gerald B. Holzman, M.D., et al., "Initial Pelvic Examination Instruction: The Effectiveness of Three Contemporary Approaches," *American Journal of Obstetrics and Gynecology* 129, no. 2 (September 15, 1977): 128.

8 Nan Robertson, "Panel Faults Breast, Pelvic Test Methods," *New York Times*, March 26, 1979.

9 See Audrey W. Mertz, "Sexual Abuse of Anesthetized Patients," in *Sexual Exploitation of Patients by Health Professionals*, ed. Ann W. Burgess, R. N., D. N.Sc., and Carol R. Hartman, R. N., D. N.Sc. (New York: Praeger, 1986), pp. 61–65. Mertz offers a case study of a male anesthesiologist "who had orally copulated with [anesthetized] women, while surgery was in process, many times during a two-year period." Nurses had reported incidences numerous times to various supervisors, but their reports had been ignored. It is interesting that in this edited volume, chapters are dedicated to anesthesiology, gynecology, and pediatrics. One could maintain that in these three specialties, patients are in particularly vulnerable positions (due to unconsciousness, youth, and direct genital contact) and the doctor-patient power differential is potentially greater than in most other specialties.

10 Not surprisingly, "Betsi," "Gynny," and "Eva" are sectioned pelvises. Unlike eighteenth-century wax models with faces, hair, and even pearls, these plastic pelvic models provide only the necessary anatomy. Perhaps this is another place in which female volition is policed. (See chapter 4 for a discussion of how sectioning and cropping function in gynecology textbook images.) For a discussion of eighteenth-century wax models, see Ludmilla Jordanova, "Body Image and Sex Roles," in *Sexual Visions: Images of Gender in Science and Medicine between the Eighteenth and Twentieth Centuries* (Madison: University of Wisconsin Press, 1989), pp. 43–65. Apparently, "dummies" were also used in American medical schools to teach medical students obstetrics. See R. W. Wertz and D. W. Wertz, *Lying-in: A History of Childbirth in America* (New Haven: Yale University Press, 1977), p. 5.

11 Dr. Robert A. Munsick uses this phrase in a discussion following Kretzschmar's article. See Kretzschmar, "Evolution," p. 373.

12 Hale and Schiner, "Professional Patients," p. 163.

13 Thomas R. Godkins, Daniel Duffy, M.D., Judith Greenwood, and William D. Stanhope, "Utilization of Simulated Patients to Teach the 'Routine' Pelvic Examination," *Journal of Medical Education* 49 (December 1974): 1175–76.

14 Buchwald, "First Pelvic Examination," p. 726.

15 I discuss this trope at length in chapter 1.

16 Godkins et al., "Utilization of Simulated Patients," p. 1177.
17 Ibid., p. 1176.
18 Kretzschmar, "Evolution," p. 368.
19 See H. S. Barrows, "The Development and Use of a New Technique in Medical Education," in *Simulated Patients (Programmed Patients)* (Springfield: Charles C. Thomas Publisher, 1971), pp. 3–42.
20 Kretzschmar, "Evolution," p. 368.
21 J. Andrew Billings, M.D., and John D. Stoekle, M.D., "Pelvic Examination Instruction and the Doctor-Patient Relationship," *Journal of Medical Education* 52 (October 1977): 838.
22 Robert M. Kretzschmar, M.D. and Deborah S. Guthrie, M.A., "Why Not in Every School?" *Journal of the American Medical Women's Association* 39, no. 2 (March/April 1984): 44.
23 Ibid.
24 C. R. B. Beckmann, M.D., et al., "Training Gynaecological Teaching Associates," *Medical Education* 22 (1988): 124. Many medical schools also employ men to teach medical students rectal and male genital exam. This program would be a fascinating topic for critical investigation.
25 Lilla A. Wallis, M.D., "The Patient as Partner in the Pelvic Exam," *The Female Patient* 7 (March 1982): 28/4–28/7. Dr. Joni Magee touched on some of Wallis's points in her important essay, "The Pelvic Examination: A View from the Other End of the Table," *Annals of Internal Medicine* 83 (1975): 563–64.
26 Wallis, "Patient as Partner," p. 28/4.
27 Arlie Russell Hochschild, *The Managed Heart: Commercialization of Human Feeling* (Berkeley: University of California Press, 1983), p. 17.
28 Traditionally, the female flight attendant's employer has regulated her in distinctly bodily ways: in addition to the demands on her emotional labor, she has been expected to strictly manage her weight and to appropriately adorn herself in terms of makeup, clothing, and heels.
29 The Women's Community Health Center, Inc. in Boston was very vocal about boycotting pelvic teaching in medical schools. See Judy Norsigian, "Training the Docs," *Health Right* (winter 1975–76): 2, 6; Women's Community Health Center, Inc., "Experiences of a Pelvic Teaching Group," *Women and Health* 1 (July/August 1976): 19–23; Susan Bell, "Political Gynecology: Gynecological Imperialism and the Politics of Self-Help," *Science for the People* (September–October 1979): 8–14. See also Wendy Barrett, Michele Dore, and Amyra Braha, "Not the Oldest Profession: Two Women Talk about Their Experiences as Professional Patients," *Healthsharing* (spring 1985): 11–14.
30 Julie M. Wilson, "The Pelvic Teaching Program at GWHC (Gainesville Women's Health Center)" *Sage-Femme* (winter 1978), p. 6.

4   Apparent Females and Female Appearances

An earlier version of this chapter appeared as "Public 'Privates' and the Gynecological Image," *Public* [8]: *The Ethics of Enactment* (1993): 184–203.
1 See Abigail Solomon-Godeau, *Photography at the Dock: Essays on Photographic History, Institutions, and Practices* (Minneapolis: University of Minnesota Press, 1990), p. 233. There are notable exceptions. For instance, see Linda Nochlin, "Courbet's *L'origine du monde*: The Origin without an Original," *October* 39 (summer 1986): 77–86.

2   In the 1970s in the United States, a medical textbook was removed from the shelves of medical libraries and discontinued due to its "pornographic" photographs of full naked bodies.

3   In medical school, students are sometimes shown mainstream porn films as part of their medical education in order to teach them about sexual activity. And as noted in chapter 3, both Louis Vontver, M.D., in the Department of Obstetrics and Gynecology, University of Washington School of Medicine, Seattle, and the University of Oklahoma Physician's Associate Program hired prostitutes to teach/model routine pelvic examination to novice students. See Thomas R. Godkins, Daniel Duffy, M.D., Judith Greenwood, and William D. Stanhope, "Utilization of Simulated Patients to Teach the 'Routine' Pelvic Examination," *Journal of Medical Education* 49 (December 1974): 1176–77.

4   AIDS activists have fought against the notion that disease is inherently unsexy. It has been critical to reconsider what is sexy in the age of AIDS. See Douglas Crimp, ed. *AIDS: Cultural Analysis, Cultural Activism* (Cambridge: MIT Press, 1987). In the edited volume, see specifically Douglas Crimp, "How to Have Promiscuity in an Epidemic," pp. 237–270.

5   James R. Scott, M.D., et al., *Danforth's Obstetrics and Gynecology*, sixth edition (Philadelphia: J. B. Lippincott Co., 1990). Since writing the majority of this chapter a seventh edition of *Danforth's* (1994) has been published. Throughout this chapter I will footnote some of the changes that have occurred between these two editions.

6   Linda Williams, *Hard Core: Power, Pleasure, and the "Frenzy of the Visible"* (Berkeley: University of California Press, 1989), p. 51.

7   Michael Lynch, "The Externalized Retina: Selection and Mathematization in the Visual Documentation of Objects in the Life Sciences," in *Representation in Scientific Practice*, ed. Michael Lynch and Steve Woolgar (Cambridge: MIT Press, 1990), p. 154.

8   Scott et al., p. 52.

9   See Thomas Laqueur, *Making Sex: Body and Gender from the Greeks to Freud* (Cambridge, Mass.: Harvard University Press, 1990). Laqueur shows that the categories of sex (male and female) are themselves historically constructed.

    Along these lines, it is a curious construction that "ambiguous genitalia" are included in an obstetrics and gynecology textbook. Why not include ambiguous genitalia in the context of male genitalia in a urology textbook? The logic for categorization is most likely due to the fact that this textbook is an obstetrics text and therefore the ambiguous genitalia of an infant should be included. However, the wedding of the ambiguous with the female is interesting.

10   The pathologization of a medically prescribed dissonance between sex (bodily materiality) and gender (bodily performance) may best be located in medical discourse about transsexuality. See Moe Meyer, "Unveiling the Word: Science and Narrative in Transsexual Striptease," *Public*[8]: *The Ethics of Enactment* (1993): 68–87. See also Sandy Stone, "The *Empire* Strikes Back: A Posttranssexual Manifesto," *Camera Obscura* 29 (1992): 151–178.

11   This image was not included in *Danforth's*, seventh edition.

12   Roland Barthes, *Image Music Text*, trans. Stephen Heath (Oxford: Oxford University Press, 1977), p. 40.

13   Julia Kristeva, *Powers of Horror: An Essay on Abjection* (New York: Columbia University Press, 1982).

14   Susan Stewart, *On Longing: Narratives of the Miniature, the Gigantic, the Souvenir, the Collection* (Durham: Duke University Press, 1993), p. 109.

15   For a collection of essays on episiotomy written by childbirth educators, midwives, and physicians, see Sheila Kitzinger and Penny Simkin, eds., *Episiotomy and the Second Stage of Labor* (Se-

attle: Pennypress, 1984). Also see John M. Thorp Jr., M.D., "Patient Autonomy, Informed Consent, and Routine Episiotomy," *Contemporary OB/Gyn* 40, no. 9 (September 1995): 92–102; Emily Martin, *The Woman in the Body: A Cultural Analysis of Reproduction*, (Boston: Beacon Press, 1987), pp. 143, 187–88.

16 M. L. Romney, "Predelivery Shaving: An Unjustified Assault?" *Journal of Obstetrics and Gynaecology* 1 (1980): pp. 33–35, cited in Ann Oakley, *Essays on Women, Medicine and Health* (Edinburgh: University of Edinburgh Press, 1993), p. 127.

17 For an important essay on contemporary Western notions of a "normal" delivery see Oakley, "Birth as a 'Normal' Process," in *Essays on Women*, pp. 124–38. See also Carol A. Stabile, "Shooting the Mother: Fetal Photography and the Politics of Disappearance," *Camera Obscura* 28, (1992): pp. 178–205.

18 This set of images has been removed from *Danforth's*, seventh edition. It has not been replaced by any other images. For that matter, there are no images of delivery or of pregnant women.

19 Roland Barthes maintains that common sense attributes pure denotation to the photograph, a utopian analogic objectivity guaranteed by its mechanical referencing of the real. See Barthes, *Image Music Text*, pp. 19, 42. But as Michael Shapiro states, "It is disclosed that representations do not imitate reality but are the practices through which things take on meaning and value; to the extent that a representation is regarded as realistic, it is because it is so familiar it operates transparently." See Shapiro, *The Politics of Representation: Writing Practices in Biography, Photography, and Policy Analysis* (Madison: University of Wisconsin Press, 1988), p. xi.

20 Johannes W. Rohen and Chihiro Yokochi, *Color Atlas of Anatomy: A Photographic Study of the Human Body* (New York: Igaku-Shoin, 1988).

21 Stewart, *On Longing*, p. 111.

22 Roland Barthes, *Camera Lucida*, trans. Richard Howard (London: Flamingo, 1981), p. 92.

23 Each of these images appears twice in *Danforth's*, seventh edition, once in a chapter titled "Physiology of Reproduction" and once in a chapter titled "Puberty and Pediatric and Adolescent Gynecology." The breast images have been renamed "Tanner Stages of Breast Development."

24 André Bazin, *What Is Cinema?* vol. 1, trans. Hugh Gray (Berkeley: University of California Press, 1967), p. 14.

25 Lisa Cartwright discusses the use of cinematic and photographic motion studies in science and medicine. See Cartwright, *Screening the Body: Tracing Medicine's Visual Culture* (Minneapolis: University of Minnesota Press, 1995), pp. 8–9, 14, 17.

26 Annette Kuhn, *The Power of the Image: Essays on Representation and Sexuality* (London: Routledge, 1985), p. 43.

27 Stewart, *On Longing*, p. 125.

28 Kaja Silverman suggests another alternative: perhaps the viewer secretly identifies with and takes pleasure in the masochistic position rather than the sadistic. Silverman particularly emphasizes the possibility of a *male* spectator's identification with the "feminine" masochistic subject position. See "Masochism and Male Subjectivity," *Camera Obscura* 17 (1988): 30–67. This idea might be especially useful when considering the male-dominated medical establishment. Though there are a progressively greater number of female clinicians, within the medical pedagogical frameworks (e.g., textbooks) I believe that the physician's subject position is still gendered male. Thus Silverman presents an underexplored aspect of male subjectivity that may be applied to the physician-patient relationship.

29 Georges Canguilhem, *The Normal and the Pathological*, trans. Carolyn R. Fawcett (New York: Zone Books, 1991), pp. 177–78.

30 Barthes, *Image Music Text*, p. 42.

31 Lynch, "The Externalized Retina," p. 162.

32 For very interesting work on visualizing technologies and science see volumes 28 and 29 of *Camera Obscura*, 1992–93, edited by Paula A. Treichler and Lisa Cartwright.

33 See Richard Dyer, "White," *Screen* 29, no. 4 (autumn 1988): 44–64.

34 This drawing has been altered in *Danforth's*, seventh edition. Now legs and buttocks are suggested in the drawing, contextualizing the viewer's perspective.

35 Daniel G. Vaughan, *General Ophthalmology*, twelfth edition (Norwalk: Appleton and Lange, 1989), p. 2. Since I first wrote this paper, the thirteenth edition of Vaughan's *General Ophthalmology* has been released. The unobscured photo of the eye has disappeared from the book's opening. Contents of medical textbooks are continually being revised, which may point to one of the limitations of close textual readings.

36 Emile A. Tanagho, M.D., and Jack W. McAninch, M.D., *Smith's General Urology*, twelfth edition (Norwalk: Appleton and Lange, 1988).

37 In a large, three-volume set titled *Campbell's Urology*, I found color plates of diseased penises comparable to those of diseased female genitalia found in *Danforth's*. Also similar to *Danforth's* was the fact that *Campbell's* provided no photographs of healthy genitals, only diagrams.

38 On the "money shot" see Williams, *Hard Core*, pp. 93–119.

39 However, when studying anatomy texts created from 1890 to 1989, researchers found that, with regard to both illustrations and descriptions, male bodies were used disproportionately as standards. In descriptions male bodies are used as the norm by which female bodies are compared. The authors found that "Modern texts . . . continue long-standing historical conventions in which male anatomy provides the basic model for 'the' human body." See Susan C. Lawrence and Kae Bendixen, "His and Hers: Male and Female Anatomy in Anatomy Texts for U.S. Medical Students 1890–1989," *Social Science and Medicine* 35, no. 7 (1992): 925–34; Kathleen D. Mendelsohn et al., "Sex and Gender Bias in Anatomy and Physical Diagnosis Text Illustrations," *Journal of the American Medical Association* 272, no. 16 (October 26, 1994): 1267–70.

40 Scott, *Danforth's*, p. 756. This image was not included in *Danforth's*, seventh edition.

41 In "Sex in Public Places: The Zaeo Aquarium Scandal and the Victorian Moral Majority," *Theater History Studies* 10 (1990), Tracy C. Davis examines the social outrage surrounding a nineteenth-century poster ad in which a gymnast, Zaeo, is pictured in a sleeveless costume with hands behind her head. This scandal was partly due to the fact that "the armpit was a Victorian metonym for female genitalia" (9). The case of Zaeo points to the historically and culturally contingent values surrounding genital, and even armpit, display.

42 "Beauty and the Beast," *The Girls of Penthouse* (March 1992).

43 The horror film is a space in which the erotics of the terrorization of women is continuously played out. But one might ask if the Beauty shown here is simultaneously the Beast. Does the voluntary display of her genitalia place her in the category of the monstrous? As will be examined in chapter 6, in David Cronenberg's *Dead Ringers* (1988) gynecology itself becomes the space of the horror (not a difficult scenario considering that many women are horrified when they visit the gynecologist). Female monstrosity is linked to internal genitalia in the incarnation of Claire Niveau, who is diagnosed as a trifurcate (possessing three cervixes that lead to three separate chambers in her uterus). For an in-depth discussion of monstrosity and the female body in horror films, see Barbara Creed, "Horror and the Monstrous-Feminine: An Imaginary Abjection," *Screen* 27, no. 1 (January–February 1986): 44–70. "Beauty and the Beast" also refers to the popular fable, most recently of Disney fame. In this story, the Beast is ugly on

the outside, while sensitive and not-so-scary on the inside. Is the Beast simply the Beauty's vulva?

44   For an interesting discussion of the beaver shot, see Kelly Dennis, " 'Leave It to Beaver': The Object of Pornography," *Strategies* 6 (1991): 122–67.

45   On early cinema and the treatment of the naked female body, see Linda Williams, "Film Body: An Implantation of Perversions," in *Narrative, Apparatus, Ideology*, ed. Philip Rosen (New York: Columbia University Press, 1986), pp. 507–34.

46   Federation of Feminist Women's Health Centers, *New View of a Woman's Body* (New York: Simon and Schuster, 1981).

47   See Luce Irigaray, *This Sex Which Is Not One*, trans. Catherine Porter (Ithaca: Cornell University Press, 1985).

48   This is evident at a historical level. For instance, medical photography has changed a great deal since its inception, when an entirely different set of codes presided. One outstanding difference was the early incorporation of patient clothes and even furniture, which effectively individualized the mise-en-scène of the pathology pictured. See Chris Amirault, "Posing the Subject of Early Medical Photography," *Discourse* 16, no. 2 (winter 1993–94): 51–76.

49   Barbara Maria Stafford, *Body Criticism: Imaging the Unseen in Enlightenment Art and Medicine* (Cambridge: MIT Press, 1991), similarly suggests that critical skills are important when making and using visual images and considers a fruitful exchange between art history and science. However, I am uncomfortable with the way Stafford rallies for the supremacy of the visual and her notion that "picture making and perception allow us to establish contact with the common somatic experience of the human race" (473).

50   In *Danforth's*, seventh edition the drawings of hysterectomies are no longer at the beginning of the text, but have been moved toward the end (p. 814). However, in Howard W. James III, M.D., Anne Colston Wentz, M.D., and Lonnie S. Burnett, M.D., *Novak's Textbook of Gynecology*, eleventh edition (Baltimore: Williams and Wilkins, 1988), the hysterectomy images also occur toward the very beginning. In a nine-hundred-page textbook, these images are found on pp. 30–34.

5   Retooling the Speculum

1   The first interview was conducted October 27, 1991, in Chicago. The second took place on June 2, 1993, in New York. I will not distinguish between the two individual interviews in this essay. The vast majority of quotes are taken from the second interview.

2   Chris Straayer, "The Seduction of Boundaries: Feminist Fluidity in Annie Sprinkle's Art/Education/Sex," in *Dirty Looks: Women, Pornography, Power*, ed. Pamela Church Gibson and Roma Gibson (London: British Film Institute, 1993): 156–75.

3   Judith Butler, *Bodies That Matter: On the Discursive Limits of "Sex"* (New York: Routledge, 1993), pp. 235–36. For an earlier discussion of drag and impersonation, see Butler, *Gender Trouble: Feminism and the Subversion of Identity* (New York: Routledge, 1989), p. 137.

4   See Sander Gilman, *Picturing Health and Illness: Images of Identity and Difference* (Baltimore: Johns Hopkins University Press, 1995).

5   Douching on stage also provides a time and place for Sprinkle to publicly urinate. Employing bodily fluids (particularly urine and female ejaculate) for transgressive and sensational performative acts will be discussed later in this chapter.

6   Barbara Creed, *The Monstrous-Feminine: Film, Feminism, Psychoanalysis* (New York: Routledge, 1993), p. 11.

7   Luce Irigaray, *Speculum of the Other Woman*, trans. Gillian C. Gill (Ithaca: Cornell University Press, 1985), p. 255. I am reminded of Sprinkle's reference to her "clean and shiny" cervix in Irigaray's discussion of this *polished* inner space of reflection.

8   Toril Moi, *Sexual/Textual Politics: Feminist Literary Theory* (London: Routledge, 1985), p. 133.

9   Irigaray, "The Blind Spot of an Old Dream of Symmetry," *Speculum*, pp. 11–129.

10 Ibid., p. 47.

12 Ibid., p. 256.

13 Shoshana Felman, "Women and Madness: The Critical Phallacy," *Diacritics* 5 (winter 1975): 3, cited in Moi, *Sexual/Textual*, p. 139.

13 See Butler, *Bodies That Matter*, p. 13. See also Eve Kosofsky Sedgwick, *Tendencies* (Durham: Duke University Press, 1993), p. 11.

14 Another performer takes an aural approach to vaginal performativity. Elizabeth Burton, an Australian performer, incorporates "pussy popping" into her striptease act. She pops along with the music by drawing air into the vagina with her muscles and then forcing it out. Her work is discussed in Lillian Lennox, "Figurations of Desire: Madame Lash, Vulvamorphia, Wicked Women" (Honor's thesis, [first class], University of Technology, Sydney, 1992).

15 On female ejaculation, see Shannon Bell, "Feminist Ejaculations," in *The Hysterical Male: New Feminist Theory*, ed. Arthur Kroker and Marilouise Kroker (New York: St. Martin's Press, 1991). Sprinkle is also a strong advocate of "Kegals," vaginal exercises during which a woman tightens her "pussy muscles" as if stopping the flow of urine. Sprinkle stresses the importance of vaginal activity over vaginal passivity for health and sexual pleasure.

16 See Georges Bataille, *Visions of Excess: Selected Writings, 1927–1939*, trans. Allan Stoekl (Minneapolis: University of Minnesota Press, 1985).

17 Mary Russo, "Female Grotesques: Carnival and Theory," in *Feminist Studies/Critical Studies*, ed. Teresa de Lauretis (Bloomington: Indiana University Press, 1986), p. 219.

18 A sentiment in line with French performance artist Orlan, whose plastic surgeries serve as performance pieces. Although critics have claimed that Orlan is simply buying into classical notions of feminine beauty, Orlan insists that her surgeries are cutting-edge critiques of such notions. At the time I saw her speak at the Performance Studies Conference at New York University, March 1995, she had made plans with Japanese surgeons to have her nose made as large as possible. Orlan intimated that this surgery would convince such critics that she was operating at a level beyond classic feminine beauty and was committed to critiquing such traditional uses of plastic surgery.

19 Linda Williams discusses legal measures taken against Sprinkle's PCA: "In 1990, while she was giving this performance in Cleveland, the municipal vice squad forced her to omit the speculum component of her act. It is a fascinating comment on American culture that when Annie Sprinkle performed live sex shows in that same city she was never visited by the vice squad." See Williams, "A Provoking Agent: The Pornography and Performance Art of Annie Sprinkle," in *Dirty Looks*, ed. Pamela Church Gibson and Roma Gibson (London: British Film Institute, 1993), p. 176.

20 Genital display and political protest have a history of camaraderie. See Lynn Hunt, *Eroticism and the Body Politic* (Baltimore: Johns Hopkins University Press, 1991). Why not cervical display?

21 See Elinor Fuchs, "Staging the Obscene Body," *Drama Review* 33 (spring 1989): 33–58.

6   Playing Doctor: Cronenberg's Surgical Construction of Mutant Female Bodies

1   Chris Rodley, ed., *Cronenberg on Cronenberg* (Boston: Faber and Faber, 1991), p. 151.

2   Walter Benjamin, "The Work of Art in the Age of Mechanical Reproduction," in *Film Theory and Criticism*, ed. Gerald Mast and Marshall Cohen (New York: Oxford University Press, 1974), p. 627.

3   Lisa Cartwright, *Screening the Body: Tracing Medicine's Visual Culture* (Minneapolis: University of Minnesota Press, 1995), p. 3.

4   It is tempting to believe, for instance, that a normal pap smear unequivocally indicates a healthy cervix. However, a pap smear is a representation, an interpretation decoded by a lab technician. It is a slide of cells, a partial perspective, and does not prove that the entire cervix is healthy.

5   Jean Baudrillard, *Simulacra and Simulation*, trans. Sheila Faria Glaser (Ann Arbor: University of Michigan Press, 1994), pp. 3–4.

6   For a discussion of endometriosis and video laparoscopy see Ella Shohat, "'Laser for Ladies': Endo Discourse and the Inscriptions of Science," *Camera Obscura* 29 (May 1992): 57–90.

7   Stephen Heath, "Narrative Space," in *Narrative, Apparatus, Ideology*, ed. Philip Rosen (New York: Columbia University Press, 1986), p. 385. For other discussions of "suture" and the cinema, see Linda Williams, "Film Body: An Implantation of Perversions," in *Narrative, Apparatus, Ideology*, p. 533 n. 4; Jaques-Alain Miller, "'Suture' (Elements of the Logic of the Signifier)," *Screen* (winter–spring 1977–1978): 24–47; Kaja Silverman, "Suture" (excerpts), in *Narrative, Apparatus, Ideology*, pp. 219–35.

8   The argument over whether Cronenberg is a true "auteur" or not as battled between Piers Handling and Robin Wood could point to the power ascribed to a cultural assembler. Cronenberg as image maker, author, and assembler of texts is a powerful person with special talents. In this sense the auteur holds a position similar to the surgeon in our culture. See Piers Handling, ed., *The Shape of Rage: The Films of David Cronenberg* (New York: New York Zoetrope, 1983).

9   Rodley, *Cronenberg on Cronenberg*, p. xii.

10   Ibid., p. 8. In fact, Cronenberg's sister, Denise Cronenberg, designed the boys' costumes after young David Cronenberg's apparel in an old family portrait.

11   Ibid., p. 145.

12   See Ludmilla Jordanova's discussion of the sculpture *Nature Unveiling Herself before Science* in *Sexual Visions: Images of Gender in Science and Medicine between the Eighteenth and Twentieth Centuries* (Madison: University of Wisconsin Press, 1989), pp. 87–110.

13   "*Dead Ringers*: Production Information" (Twentieth Century Fox Film Corporation, 1988), p. 3.

14   Mary Russo provides a different take on Claire's relationship to the public and private in her thought-provoking chapter on *Dead Ringers*. She remarks on Claire's "seeming invulnerability to intimidation by the doctors in the actual exposure of her vagina and her *extreme* vulnerability to *public* exposure of her internal abnormality because she is an actress, a professional woman. In other words, the usual public/private distinctions are reversed and even untenable for the actress" (pp. 119–20). See Russo, "Twins and Mutant Women: David Cronenberg's *Dead Ringers*," in *The Female Grotesque: Risk, Excess and Modernity* (New York: Routledge, 1995), pp. 107–127.

15   Sigmund Freud, "Medusa's Head," *Standard Edition*, trans. James Strachey (London: Hogarth, 1953–66), 18: 273–74.

16   Andrew Parker cleverly refers to Rose's protrusion as "a penis *dentatus*." See Parker, "Grafting

David Cronenberg: Monstrosity, AIDS Media, National/Sexual Difference," *Stanford Humanities Review* 3, no. 1 (winter 1993): 11.

17   For a delightfully unpsychoanalytic but problematically celebratory account of Cronenberg's work, see Steven Shaviro, "Bodies of Fear: David Cronenberg," in *The Cinematic Body* (Minneapolis: University of Minnesota Press, 1993), pp. 127–56.

18   Thomas Laqueur, *Making Sex: Body and Gender from the Greeks to Freud* (Cambridge, Mass.: Harvard University Press, 1990), p. 89.

19   Ibid., p. 34.

20   Carol Clover suggests, "Horror may in fact be the premier repository of one-sex reasoning in our time (science fiction running a close second)." Clover, however, links one-sex reasoning to Freud, using his ideas of penis envy, phallic women, and anal menstruation/intercourse/birth as evidence. Thus for Clover psychoanalysis and one-sex reasoning can work together. Cronenberg's films, including *Dead Ringers*, are located across the genres of both horror and sci-fi. Cronenberg's use of the Rueff image may be the most overt and historic reference to one-sex reasoning in his films. See Clover, *Men, Women, and Chainsaws: Gender in the Modern Horror Film* (Princeton: Princeton University Press, 1992).

21   See Barbara Creed's "Phallic Panic: Male Hysteria and *Dead Ringers*," *Screen* (summer 1990): 125–46. This essay is an excellent exploration of castration anxiety in this film.

22   Luce Irigaray, *This Sex Which Is Not One*, trans. Catherine Porter (Ithaca: Cornell University Press, 1985), p. 26.

23   Rodley, *Cronenberg on Cronenberg*, p. 196.

24   Elaine Showalter, *The Female Malady: Women, Madness, and English Culture, 1830–1980* (New York: Penguin, 1985), p. 156.

25   Freud, "Hysteria," *Standard Edition*, 1:43.

26   Ibid., 1:52.

27   Mary Poovey, "'Scenes of an Indelicate Character': The Medical 'Treatment' of Victorian Women," *Representations* 14 (spring 1986): 153.

28   One woman I spoke with had been referred by a physician to a prominent gynecologist at a major hospital in Chicago in order to evaluate her PMS. When she told him about her PMS and how it made her feel horrible and crazy, he explained that he could not suggest birth control pills because these hadn't seemed to help other patients. She asked him what he could suggest. He replied, "I know a good psychiatrist I can refer you to." The uterus, its "malfunction," causes performative outbreaks that can only be treated by a psychiatrist. These notions are still common today.

29   The answer is undoubtedly "no," as the male assistant is coded as gay and appears repulsed by any suggestion of physical intimacy with Claire.

30   Russo, *Female Grotesque*, p. 108.

31   Creed, "Phallic Panic," p. 142.

32   Robin Wood has criticized Cronenberg for believing that his films do not have an ideology. Wood is enraged by Cronenberg's belief that his works reside outside political criticism. See Wood, "Cronenberg: A Dissenting View," in *The Shape of Rage: The Films of David Cronenberg*, ed. Piers Handling (New York: New York Zoetrope, 1983), pp. 115–35.

33   Joan Copjec, "Cinematic Pleasure and Sexual Difference: The Delirium of Clinical Perfection," *Oxford Literary Review* 8, nos. 1–2 (1986): 57.

34   Anne Billson, "Cronenberg on Cronenberg: A Career in Stereo," *Monthly Film Bulletin* 56, no. 660 (January 1989): 3–6.

35   The theatricality of gynecology is evident in Cronenberg's staging of gynecological surgery: the operating team is costumed in blood-red gowns as though they are participating in a religious pageant.

36   Similarly, Andrew Parker suggests that Cronenberg's *Rabid* adds to the discourse on AIDS mania. However, *Rabid* preceded AIDS awareness and thus Parker suggests a more unidirectional transferal of meaning than I am suggesting here with regard to *Dead Ringers* and gynecological practice. Parker writes, "Should we infer that Cronenberg was unconsciously prophetic, that he 'knew' in advance how AIDS will have been constructed? I am, of course, hardly claiming that. The point, rather, runs in the opposite direction, for the mainstream media response to AIDS has taken its representational bearings from pre-existing, culturally pervasive 'narrative systems' . . . " ("Grafting," p. 12).

37   Pete Boss, "Vile Bodies and Bad Medicine," *Screen* 27 (1986): 16.

38   A friend of mine who enjoyed Cronenberg's *Rabid* had never seen *Dead Ringers*. When I suggested that she view it she replied, "I think I'll wait. I'm due for a pap smear soon."

39   For a fascinating account of the association of gynecology with sex and violence in Victorian times see Coral Lansbury, "Gynaecology, Pornography, and the Antivivisection Movement," *Victorian Studies* 28 (spring 1985): 413–37.

7   *The Other End of the Speculum*

1   Over the course of six years (1990–96), I have interviewed over three hundred women in Chicago who have experienced a variety of gynecological practices.

2   Federation of Feminist Women's Health Centers, *New View of a Woman's Body* (New York: Simon and Schuster, 1981), p. 19.

3   Ronnie Lichtman, C.N.M., M.S., M.Phil., and Susan Papera, C.N.M., M.S., eds., *Gynecology: Well-Woman Care* (East Norwalk, Conn.: Appleton and Lange, 1990), p. xiv.

4   Boston Women's Health Book Collective, *The New Our Bodies, Ourselves* (New York: Simon and Schuster, 1992), p. 677.

5   On menstrual extraction, see Rebecca Salstrom, "Menstrual Extraction: Is Self Help Making a Comeback?" *Women Wise* 15, no. 1 (1992): 2–4.

6   Donna J. Haraway, *Simians, Cyborgs, and Women: The Reinvention of Nature* (New York: Routledge, 1991), p. 169.

7   Stephen Grosz and Bruce McAuley, "*Self-Health* and *Healthcaring*," *Camera Obscura* 7 (1981): 131.

8   Onlywomen Health Group, "Down There," *Spare Rib*, 52, n.d.

9   See "Vulvar Self Exam," *Modern Medicine* 58 (February 1990): 30–31.

10   Paula A. Treichler and Lisa Cartwright, eds., *Camera Obscura* 28 (1992): 8.

11   Haraway, *Simians, Cyborgs, and Women*, p. 198.

12   See Walt Bogdanich, *The Great White Lie: Dishonesty, Waste, and Incompetence in the Medical Community* (New York: Touchstone, 1991); George C. Halvorson, *Strong Medicine* (New York: Random House, 1993); Dave Lindorff, *Marketplace Medicine: The Rise of the For-Profit Hospital Chains* (New York: Bantam, 1992); Nancy F. McKenzie, ed., *Beyond Crisis: Confronting Health Care in the United States* (New York: Meridian, 1994); Lawrence D. Weiss, *No Benefit: Crisis in America's Health Insurance Industry* (Boulder: Westview, 1992).

13   As an experiment one University of Chicago student made numerous calls to the university's

gynecology clinic claiming his wife needed an appointment: "When I told the clinic my wife had Blue Cross insurance, she was given an appointment for October 18 with no wait, was offered the choice of seeing a male or female doctor, and was told the name of the doctor she would be seeing. When the insurance was Medicaid, I was left on hold for three minutes, was neither asked if she preferred a male or female doctor nor told her doctor's name. I was given an appointment at the clinic—on November 29, well over a month later than the appointment I was given with Blue Cross." See J. W. Mason, "Double Standard," *The Nation* (January 9/16, 1995): 52. See also Laurie Kaye Abraham, *Mama Might Be Better Off Dead: The Failure of Health Care in Urban America* (Chicago: University of Chicago Press, 1994).

14 Bonnie J. Kay, "The Commodification of Women's Health: The New Women's Health Centers," *Health/ PAC Bulletin* (winter 1989): 19–23.

15 Joan P. Emerson, "Behavior in Private Places: Sustaining Definitions of Reality in Gynecological Examination," in *Recent Sociology No. 2: Patterns of Communicative Behavior*, ed. Hans Peter Dreitzel (London: Macmillan, 1970), p. 78.

16 On the role of the health worker, see Vicki L. Smith, "Sharing Ourselves . . . Our Greatest Strength," *Women Wise* 9, no. 2 (summer 1986): 6–7; and Pat Moran, "I Am a Feminist Healthworker . . . Still," *Women Wise* 9, no. 2 (summer 1986): 7.

17 Stephen A. Tyler, *The Unspeakable: Discourse, Dialogue, and Rhetoric in the Postmodern World* (Madison: University of Wisconsin Press, 1987), p. 157.

18 George Lakoff and Mark Johnson, *Metaphors We Live By* (Chicago: University of Chicago Press, 1980), p. 194.

19 Michael Taussig, *Mimesis and Alterity: A Particular History of the Senses* (New York: Routledge, 1993), p. 21.

20 Ibid., p. 25.

21 Eve Kosofsky Sedgwick notes, "anxiety about girls' and women's masturbation contributed more to the emergence of gynecology, through an accumulated expertise in and demand for genital surgery . . . Far from there persisting a minority identity of 'the masturbator' today, of course, autoeroticism per se in the twentieth century has been conclusively subsumed under that normalizing developmental model, differently but perhaps equally demeaning, according to which it represents a relatively innocuous way station on the road to a 'full,' i.e., alloerotic, adult genitality defined almost exclusively by gender of the object choice." Though masturbation is no longer "treated" through gynecological surgery in this country, it is still far from "innocuous." See Sedgwick, "Jane Austen and the Masturbating Girl," in *Tendencies* (Durham: Duke University Press, 1993), p. 117.

22 Theater theorist Jill Dolan states, "Deconstructing the performance apparatus in postmodernist terms is not politically progressive unless the gender assumptions that underlie representation are also denaturalized and changed." She notes progress when more women are relegated to "authoritative positions" in the theater (e.g., director). However, what is left uncritiqued is that these very authoritative positions (director or, for instance, physician) serve to fortify structures within the apparatus that are both naturalized and gendered. See Dolan, *Feminist Spectator as Critic* (Ann Arbor: UMI Research, 1988), p. 16.

Bibliography

Abraham, Laurie Kaye. *Mama Might Be Better Off Dead: The Failure of Health Care in Urban America*. Chicago: University of Chicago Press, 1994.

Altick, Richard Daniel. *The Shows of London*. Cambridge, Mass.: Harvard University Press, 1978.

American Health Consultants. "Clinicians, Patients, Medicaid: Is Anyone to Blame for Norplant Removal Dilemma?" *Contraceptive Technology Update* 14, no. 10 (October 1993): 149–53.

———. "Too Much or Too Little: Access to Norplant Implants Fuels Ethics Debate." *Contraceptive Technology Update* 14, no. 9 (September 1993): 133–36.

Amirault, Chris. "Posing the Subject of Early Medical Photography." *Discourse* 16, no. 2 (winter 1993–94): 51–76.

Arthur, Stacey L. "The Norplant Prescription: Birth Control, Woman Control, or Crime Control?" *UCLS Law Review* 40, no. 1 (1992): 1–101.

Axelsen, Diana E. "Women as Victims of Medical Experimentation: J. Marion Sims' Surgery on Slave Women, 1845–50." *Sage* 2, no. 2 (fall 1985): 10–13.

Bakhtin, Mikhail. *Rabelais and His World*. Translated by Helene Iswolsky. Bloomington: Indiana University Press, 1984.

Baldwin, W. O. "Tribute to the Late James Marion Sims, November, 1883." In *The Story of My Life*. By J. Marion Sims, M.D. New York: D. Appleton and Company, 1886.

Barker-Benfield, G. J. *The Horrors of the Half-Known Life*. New York: Harper & Row, 1976.

Barrett, Wendy, Michele Dore, and Amyra Braha. "Not the Oldest Profession: Two Women Talk about Their Experiences as Professional Patients." *Healthsharing* (spring 1985): 11–14.

Barrows, H. S. *Simulated Patients (Programmed Patients)*. Springfield: Charles C. Thomas Publisher, 1971.

Barthes, Roland. *Camera Lucida*. Translated by Richard Howard. London: Flamingo, 1981.

————. *Image Music Text*. Translated by Stephen Heath. Oxford: Oxford University Press, 1977.

Bataille, Georges. *Visions of Excess: Selected Writings, 1927–1939*. Translated by Allan Stoekl. Minneapolis: University of Minnesota Press, 1985.

Baudrillard, Jean. *Simulacra and Simulation*. Translated by Sheila Faria Glaser. Ann Arbor: University of Michigan Press, 1994.

Baudry, Jean-Louis. "Ideological Effects of the Basic Cinematographic Apparatus." In *Narrative, Apparatus, Ideology*. Edited by Philip Rosen. New York: Columbia University Press, 1988, pp. 286–98.

Bazin, André. *What Is Cinema?* Vol. 1. Translated by Hugh Gray. Berkeley: University of California Press, 1967.

"Beauty and the Beast." *The Girls of Penthouse* (March 1992).

Beckmann, M.D., C. R. B., et al. "Training Gynaecological Teaching Associates." *Medical Education* 22 (1988): 124–31.

Bell, Shannon. "Feminist Ejaculations." In *The Hysterical Male: New Feminist Theory*. Edited by Arthur Kroker and Marilouise Kroker. New York: St. Martin's Press, 1991, pp. 155–69.

Bell, Susan. "Political Gynecology: Gynecological Imperialism and the Politics of Self-Help." *Science for the People* (September–October 1979): 8–14.

Benjamin, Walter. "The Work of Art in the Age of Mechanical Reproduction." In *Film Theory and Criticism*. Edited by Gerald Mast and Marshall Cohen. New York: Oxford University Press, 1974, pp. 612–34.

Bergstrom, Janet, and Mary Ann Doane, eds. *Camera Obscura* 20–21 (May–September 1989).

Billings, M.D., J. Andrew, and John D. Stoekle, M.D. "Pelvic Examination Instruction and the Doctor-Patient Relationship." *Journal of Medical Education* 52 (October 1977): 834–39.

Billson, Anne. "Cronenberg on Cronenberg: A Career in Stereo." *Monthly Film Bulletin* 56, no. 660 (January 1989): 3–6.

Blount, Melissa. "Surpassing Obstacles: Pioneering Black Women Physicians." In *The Black Women's Health Book: Speaking for Ourselves*. Edited by Evelyn C. White. Seattle: Seal Press, 1990, pp. 44–51.

Bogdanich, Walt. *The Great White Lie: Dishonesty, Waste, and Incompetence in the Medical Community*. New York: Touchstone, 1991.

Boss, Pete. "Vile Bodies and Bad Medicine." *Screen* 27, no. 1 (1986): 14–24.

Boston Women's Health Book Collective. *The New Our Bodies, Ourselves*. New York: Simon and Schuster, 1992.

Bruno, Giuliana. "Spectatorial Embodiments: Anatomies of the Visible and the Female Bodyscape." *Camera Obscura* 28 (January 1992): 239–61.

Buchwald, M.D., Julius. "The First Pelvic Examination: Helping Students Cope with Their Emotional Reactions." *Journal of Medical Education* 54 (September 1979): 725–28.

Butler, Judith. *Bodies That Matter: On the Discursive Limits of "Sex."* New York: Routledge, 1993.

————. *Gender Trouble: Feminism and the Subversion of Identity*. New York: Routledge, 1989.

Byford, Henry T. *Manual of Gynecology*. Philadelphia: P. Blakiston, Son and Co., 1897.

Canguilhem, Georges. *The Normal and the Pathological*. Translated by Carolyn R. Fawcett. New York: Zone Books, 1991.

Carby, Hazel. *Reconstructing Womanhood: The Emergence of the Afro-American Woman Novelist*. New York: Oxford University Press, 1987.

Cartwright, Lisa. *Screening the Body: Tracing Medicine's Visual Culture*. Minneapolis: University of Minnesota Press, 1995.

Clover, Carol J. *Men, Women, and Chainsaws: Gender in the Modern Horror Film*. Princeton: Princeton University Press, 1992.

Copjec, Joan. "Cinematic Pleasure and Sexual Difference: The Delirium of Clinical Perfection." *Oxford Literary Review* 8, nos. 1–2 (1986): 57–65.

Creed, Barbara. *The Monstrous-Feminine: Film, Feminism, Psychoanalysis*. London: Routledge, 1993.

———. "Phallic Panic: Male Hysteria and *Dead Ringers*."*Screen* (summer 1990): 125–46.

———. "Horror and the Monstrous-Feminine: An Imaginary Abjection." *Screen* 27, no. 1 (January–February 1986): 44–70.

Crimp, Douglas, ed. *AIDS: Cultural Analysis, Cultural Activism*. Cambridge: MIT Press, 1987.

Davis, Angela. "The Black Woman's Role in the Community of Slaves." *Black Scholar* 3 (December 1971): 2.

Davis, Sheila P., and Cora A. Ingram. "Empowered Caretakers: A Historical Perspective on the Roles of Granny Midwives in Rural Alabama." In *Wings of Gauze: Women of Color and the Experience of Health and Illness*. Edited by Barbara Bair and Susan E. Cayleff. Detroit: Wayne State University Press, 1993, pp. 191–201.

Davis, Tracy C. "Sex in Public Places: The Zaeo Aquarium Scandal and the Victorian Moral Majority." *Theater History Studies* 10 (1990): 1–13.

Davy, Kate. "Fe-Male Impersonation: The Discourse of Camp." In *Politics and Poetics of Camp*. Edited by Moe Meyer. New York: Routledge, 1994, pp. 130–48.

"*Dead Ringers*: Production Information." Twentieth Century Fox Film Corporation, 1988.

deCerteau, Michel. *Practice of Everyday Life*. Translated by Steven Rendall. Berkeley: University of California Press, 1984.

de Lauretis, Teresa. *Alice Doesn't: Feminism, Semiotics, Cinema*. Bloomington: Indiana University Press, 1984.

———. *Technologies of Gender*. Bloomington: Indiana University Press, 1987.

D'Emilio, John, and Estelle B. Freedman. *Intimate Matters: A History of Sexuality in America*. New York: Harper & Row, 1988.

Dennis, Kelly. "'Leave It to Beaver': The Object of Pornography." *Strategies* 6 (1991): 122–67.

Diamond, Elin. "Brechtian Theory/Feminist Theory: Toward a Gestic Feminist Criticism." *The Drama Review* 32, no. 1 (1988): 82–94.

Doane, Mary Ann. *Femmes Fatales: Feminism, Film Theory, Psychoanalysis*. New York: Routledge, 1991.

———. *The Desire to Desire*. Bloomington: Indiana University Press, 1987.

Dolan, Jill. *Presence and Desire*. Ann Arbor: University of Michigan Press, 1993.

———. *Feminist Spectator as Critic*. Ann Arbor: UMI Research, 1988.

Doty, Alexander. *Making Things Perfectly Queer: Interpreting Mass Culture*. Minneapolis: University of Minnesota Press, 1993.

Douglas, Mary. *Purity and Danger: An Analysis of Concepts of Pollution and Taboo*. London: Routledge, 1966.

Drewal, Margaret Thompson. "From Rocky's Rockettes to Liberace: The Politics of Representation in the Heart of Corporate Capitalism." *Journal of American Culture* 10, no. 2 (summer 1987): 69–82.

Dyer, Richard. "White." *Screen* 29, no. 4 (autumn 1988): 44–64.

———, ed. *Gays in Film* (London: BFI, 1980).

Ehrenreich, Barbara, and Deirdre English. *For Her Own Good: 150 Years of the Experts' Advice to Women*. New York: Doubleday, 1978.

Emerson, Joan P. "Behavior in Private Places: Sustaining Definitions of Reality in Gynecological Examinations." In *Recent Sociology No. 2: Patterns of Communicative Behavior*. Edited by Hans Peter Dreitzel. London: Macmillan, 1970, pp. 74–97.

Federation of Feminist Women's Health Centers. *New View of a Woman's Body*. New York: Simon and Schuster, 1981.

Felman, Shoshana. "Women and Madness: The Critical Phallacy." *Diacritics* 5 (winter 1975): 2–5.

Foucault, Michel. *The Birth of the Clinic: An Archaeology of Medical Perception*. Translated by A. M. Sheridan Smith. New York: Random House, 1973.

———. *Power/Knowledge: Selected Interviews and Other Writings 1972–1977*. Edited by Colin Gordon. New York: Pantheon, 1972.

Fox-Genovese, Elizabeth. *Within the Plantation Household: Black and White Women of the South*. Chapel Hill: University of North Carolina Press, 1988.

Freud, Sigmund. "Medusa's Head." *The Standard Edition of the Complete Psychological Works of Sigmund Freud*. 24 vols. Translated by James Strachey. London: Hogarth, 1953–66, 18: 273–74.

———. "Hysteria." *The Standard Edition of the Complete Psychological Works of Sigmund Freud*. 24 vols. Translated by James Strachey. London: Hogarth, 1953–66, 1:41–57.

Fuchs, Elinor. "Staging the Obscene Body." *Drama Review* 33 (spring 1989): 33–58.

Gamman, Lorraine, and Margaret Marshment, eds. *The Female Gaze: Women as Viewers of Popular Culture*. Seattle: Real Comet Press, 1989.

Gilbert, Susan. "Bias in Doctors' Offices May Harm Gay Women's Health, Study Finds." *New York Times*, October 11, 1995.

Gilman, Sander. *Picturing Health and Illness: Images of Identity and Difference*. Baltimore: Johns Hopkins University Press, 1995.

———. *Difference and Pathology: Stereotypes of Sex, Race, and Madness*. Ithaca: Cornell University Press, 1985.

———. "Black Bodies, White Bodies: Toward an Iconography of Female Sexuality in Late Nineteenth-Century Art, Medicine, and Literature." *Critical Inquiry* (autumn 1985): 204–42.

Godkins, Thomas R., Daniel Duffy, M.D., Judith Greenwood, and William D. Stanhope. "Utilization of Simulated Patients to Teach the 'Routine' Pelvic Examination." *Journal of Medical Education* 49 (December 1974): 1174–78.

Grosz, Stephen, and Bruce McAuley. "*Self-Health* and *Healthcaring*." *Camera Obscura* 7 (1981): 129–35.

Hale, M.D., Ralph W., and Wilma Schiner, R.N. "Professional Patients: An Improved Method of Teaching Breast and Pelvic Examination." *Journal of Reproductive Medicine* 19, no. 3 (September 1977): 163–66.

Halvorson, George C. *Strong Medicine*. New York: Random House, 1993.

Haraway, Donna J. *Simians, Cyborgs, and Women: The Reinvention of Nature*. New York: Routledge, 1991.

Harris, M.D., Seale. *Woman's Surgeon: The Life Story of J. Marion Sims*. New York: Macmillan, 1950.

Hartmann, Betsey. *Reproductive Rights and Wrongs: The Global Politics of Population Control and Contraceptive Choice*. New York: Harper & Row, 1987.

Hatcher, M.D., M.P.H., Robert A., et al. *Contraceptive Technology*. 15th rev. ed. New York: Irvington, 1994.

Heath, Stephen. "Narrative Space." In *Narrative, Apparatus, Ideology*. Edited by Philip Rosen. New York: Columbia University Press, 1986, pp. 379–420.

Henslin, James M., and Mae A. Biggs. "Dramaturgical Desexualization: The Sociology of Vaginal Examination." In *Studies in the Sociology of Sex*. Edited by James M. Henslin. New York: Appleton-Century-Crofts, 1971, pp. 243–72.

Hine, Darlene Clark. "Mabel K. Stauper and the Integration of Black Nurses into the Armed Forces." In *Women and Health in America*. Edited by Judith Walzer Leavitt. Madison: University of Wisconsin Press, 1984, pp. 497–506.

Hochschild, Arlie Russell. *The Managed Heart: Commercialization of Human Feeling*. Berkeley: University of California Press, 1983.

Holzman, M.D., Gerald B., et al. "Initial Pelvic Examination Instruction: The Effectiveness of Three Contemporary Approaches." *American Journal of Obstetrics and Gynecology* 129, no. 2 (September 15, 1977): 124–31.

Hunt, Lynn. *Eroticism and the Body Politic*. Baltimore: Johns Hopkins University Press, 1991.

Irigaray, Luce. *Speculum of the Other Woman*. Translated by Gillian C. Gill. Ithaca: Cornell University Press, 1985.

———. *This Sex Which Is Not One*. Translated by Catherine Porter. Ithaca: Cornell University Press, 1985.

James III M.D., Howard W., Anne Colston Wentz, M.D., and Lonnie S. Burnett, M.D., eds. *Novak's Textbook of Gynecology*. 11th ed. Baltimore: Williams and Wilkins, 1988.

Jones, James H. *Bad Blood: The Tuskegee Syphilis Experiment*. New York: Free Press, 1993.

Jones, Lisa. *Bulletproof Diva: Tales of Race, Sex, and Hair*. New York: Anchor Books, 1994.

Jordan, Winthrop D. *White over Black: American Attitudes toward the Negro, 1550–1812*. New York: W. W. Norton, 1968.

Jordanova, Ludmilla. *Sexual Visions: Images of Gender in Science and Medicine between the Eighteenth and Twentieth Centuries*. Madison: University of Wisconsin Press, 1989.

Juno, Andrea, and V. Vale, eds. *Angry Women*. San Francisco: Re/Search Publications, 1991.

Kaiser, M.D., Irwin H. "Reappraisals of J. Marion Sims." *American Journal of Obstetrics and Gynecology* 132 (1978): 878–84.

Kay, Bonnie J. "The Commodification of Women's Health: The New Women's Health Centers." *Health/PAC Bulletin* (winter 1989): 19–23.

King, Thomas A. "Performing 'Akimbo': Queer Pride and Epistemological Prejudice." In *Politics and Poetics of Camp*. Edited by Moe Meyer. New York: Routledge, 1994, pp. 23–50.

Kipnis, Laura. *Ecstasy Unlimited: On Sex, Capital, Gender, and Aesthetics*. Minneapolis: University of Minnesota Press, 1993.

Kitzinger, Sheila, and Penny Simkin, eds. *Episiotomy and the Second Stage of Labor*. Seattle: Pennypress, 1984.

Kretzschmar, M.D., Robert M. "Evolution of the Gynecology Teaching Associate: An Education Specialist." *American Journal of Obstetrics and Gynecology* 131, no. 4 (June 15, 1978): 367–73.

Kretzschmar, M.D., Robert M., and Deborah S. Guthrie, M.A. "Why Not in Every School?" *Journal of the American Medical Women's Association* 39, no. 2 (March/April 1984): 43–45.

Kristeva, Julia. *Powers of Horror: An Essay on Abjection*. New York: Columbia University Press, 1982.

Kuhn, Annette. *The Power of the Image: Essays on Representation and Sexuality*. London: Routledge, 1985.

Lakoff, George, and Mark Johnson. *Metaphors We Live By*. Chicago: University of Chicago Press, 1980.

Lansbury, Coral. "Gynaecology, Pornography, and the Antivivisection Movement." *Victorian Studies* 28 (spring 1985): 413–37.

Laqueur, Thomas. *Making Sex: Body and Gender from the Greeks to Freud*. Cambridge, Mass.: Harvard University Press, 1990.

Lawrence, Susan C., and Kae Bendixen. "His and Hers: Male and Female Anatomy in Anatomy Texts for U.S. Medical Students 1890–1989." *Social Science and Medicine* 35, no. 7 (1992): 925–34.

Lennox, Lillian. "Figurations of Desire: Madame Lash, Vulvamorphia, Wicked Women." Honor's thesis (first class), University of Technology, Sydney, 1992.

Lewin, Tamar. "Baltimore School Clinics to Offer Birth Control by Surgical Implant." *New York Times*, December 4, 1992.

Lichtman, C.N.M., M.S., M.Phil., Ronnie, and Susan Papera, C.N.M., M.S., eds. *Gynecology: Well-Woman Care*. East Norwalk, Conn.: Appleton and Lange, 1990.

Lindorff, Dave. *Marketplace Medicine: The Rise of the For-Profit Hospital Chains*. New York: Bantam, 1992.

Little, Heather M. "No Panacea: Norplant Suit Charges Failure to Educate Patients." *Chicago Tribune*, October 31, 1993.

Long, Gretchen. "Norplant: A Victory, Not a Panacea for Poverty." *The National Lawyers Guild Practitioner* 50, no. 1 (winter 1993): 11–13.

Longo, Lawrence D. "The Rise and Fall of Battey's Operation: A Fashion in Surgery." In *Women and Health in America*. Edited by Judith Walzer Leavitt. Madison: University of Wisconsin Press, 1984, pp. 270–84.

Lynch, Michael. "The Externalized Retina: Selection and Mathematization in the Visual Documentation of Objects in the Life Sciences." In *Representation in Scientific Practice*. Edited by Michael Lynch and Steve Woolgar. Cambridge: MIT Press, 1990, pp. 153–86.

Magee, M.D., Joni. "The Pelvic Examination: A View from the Other End of the Table." *Annals of Internal Medicine* 83 (1975): 563–64.

Martin, Emily. *The Woman in the Body: A Cultural Analysis of Reproduction*. Boston: Beacon Press, 1987.

Mason, J. W. "Double Standard." *The Nation* (January 9/16, 1995): 52.

Mayne, Judith. *Cinema and Spectatorship*. New York: Routledge, 1993.

McKenzie, Nancy F., ed. *Beyond Crisis: Confronting Health Care in the United States*. New York: Meridian, 1994.

Mendelsohn, Kathleen D., et al. "Sex and Gender Bias in Anatomy and Physical Diagnosis Text Illustrations." *Journal of the American Medical Association* 272, no. 16 (October 26, 1994): 1267–70.

Mertz, Audrey W. "Sexual Abuse of Anesthetized Patients." In *Sexual Exploitation of Patients by Health Professionals*. Edited by Ann W. Burgess, R.N., D.N.Sc., and Carol R. Hartman, R.N., D.N.Sc. New York: Praeger, 1986, pp. 61–65.

Metz, Christian. "The Imaginary Signifier [Excerpts]." In *Narrative, Apparatus, Ideology*. Edited by Philip Rosen. New York: Columbia University Press, 1986, pp. 244–78.

Meyer, Moe. "Unveiling the Word: Science and Narrative in Transsexual Striptease." *Public 8: The Ethics of Enactment* (1993): 68–87.

Miller, Jaques-Alain. "'Suture' (Elements of the Logic of the Signifier)." *Screen* 18 (winter–spring 1977–1978): 24–47.

Mintzes, Barbara, Anita Hardon, and Jannemieke Hanhart, eds. *Norplant: Under Her Skin*. Amsterdam: Women's Health Action Foundation, 1993.

Mitford, Jessica. *The American Way of Birth*. New York: Dutton, 1992.

Moi, Toril. *Sexual/Textual Politics: Feminist Literary Theory*. London: Routledge, 1985.

Moir, J. Chassar. *The Vesico-Vaginal Fistula*. 2d ed. London: Bailliere Tindall and Cassell, 1967.

Montano, Linda. *Art in Everyday Life*. New York: Station Hill, 1981.

Moran, Pat. "I Am a Feminist Healthworker . . . Still." *Women Wise* 9, no. 2 (summer 1986): 7.

Morrow, Shana. "Welfare Reform and Reproductive Freedom." *Planned Parenthood Chicago Area: Political Affairs Perspective* (fall 1993): 2–3, 7.

Mulvey, Laura. *Visual and Other Pleasures*. Bloomington: Indiana University Press, 1989.

————. "Visual Pleasure and Narrative Cinema." *Screen* 16, no. 3 (autumn 1975): 6–18.

National Black Women's Health Project. "Facts: Norplant" (newsletter), 1992.

Native American Women's Health Education Resource Center. "Native American Women Uncover Norplant Abuses." *Ms.* (September/October 1993): 69.

————. *The Impact of Norplant in the Native American Community*, Native American Women's Health Education Resource Center, 1992.

Nead, Lynda. *The Female Nude: Art, Obscenity and Sexuality*. London: Routledge, 1992.

Nochlin, Linda. "Courbet's *L'origine du monde*: The Origin without an Original." *October* 39 (summer 1986): 77–86.

Norsigian, Judy. "Training the Docs." *Health Right* 2 (winter 1975–76): 2, 6.

Oakley, Ann. *Essays on Women, Medicine and Health*. Edinburgh: University of Edinburgh Press, 1993.

Ojanuga, Durrenda. "The Medical Ethics of the 'Father of Gynaecology,' Dr. J. Marion Sims." *Journal of Medical Ethics* 19 (1993): 28–31.

Ollila, Eeva, Kristiina Kajesalo, and Elina Hemminki. "Experience of Norplant by Finnish Family Planning Practitioners." In *Norplant: Under Her Skin*. Edited by Barbara Mintzes, Anita Hardon, and Jannemieke Hanhart. Amsterdam: Women's Health Action Foundation, 1993, pp. 47–68.

Onlywomen Health Group. "Down There." *Spare Rib* n.d.: 52–55.

Parker, Andrew. "Grafting David Cronenberg: Monstrosity, AIDS Media, National/Sexual Difference." *Stanford Humanities Review* 3, no. 1 (winter 1993): 7–19.

Pear, Robert. "Population Growth Outstrips Earlier U.S. Census Estimates." *New York Times*, December 4, 1992.

Phelan, Peggy. *Unmarked: The Politics of Performance*. New York: Routledge, 1993.

Poovey, Mary. "'Scenes of an Indelicate Character': The Medical 'Treatment' of Victorian Women." *Representations* 14 (spring 1986): 137–68.

The Population Council. *Norplant Worldwide* 16 (November 1991).

Pribram, E. Deidre, ed. *Female Spectators: Looking at Film and Television*. London: Verso, 1988.

Purvis, A. "A Pill That Gets under the Skin. Norplant Could Spur Birth Control—and Stir Controversy." *Time* (December 24, 1990): 45.

Roberts, Dorothy E. "Crime, Race, and Reproduction." *Tulane Law Review* 67 (1993): 1945–77.

Robertson, Nan. "Panel Faults Breast, Pelvic Test Methods." *New York Times*, March 26, 1979.

Rodley, Chris, ed. *Cronenberg on Cronenberg*. Boston: Faber and Faber, 1991.

Rohen, Johannes W., and Chihiro Yokochi. *Color Atlas of Anatomy: A Photographic Study of the Human Body*. New York: Igaku-Shoin, 1988.

Romney, M. L. "Predelivery Shaving: An Unjustified Assault?" *Journal of Obstetrics and Gynaecology* 1 (1980): 33–35.

Rosen, Philip, ed. *Narrative, Apparatus, Ideology*. New York: Columbia University Press, 1988.

Rosser, Sue V. *Women's Health: Missing from U.S. Medicine*. Bloomington: University of Indiana Press, 1994.

Russo, Mary. *The Female Grotesque: Risk, Excess and Modernity*. New York: Routledge, 1995.

————. "Female Grotesques: Carnival and Theory." In *Feminist Studies/Critical Studies*. Edited by Teresa de Lauretis. Bloomington: Indiana University Press, 1986.

Salstrom, Rebecca. "Menstrual Extraction: Is Self Help Making a Comeback?" *Women Wise* 15, no. 1 (1992): 2–4.

Savitt, Todd L. "Black Health on the Plantation: Masters, Slaves, and Physicians." In *Science and Medicine in the Old South*. Edited by Ronald L. Numbers and Todd L. Savitt. Baton Rouge: Louisiana State University Press, 1989: 327–55.

———. "The Use of Blacks for Medical Experimentation and Demonstration in the Old South." *The Journal of Southern History* 48, no. 3 (August 1982): 273–347.

———. *Medicine and Slavery: The Diseases and Health Care of Blacks in Ante-bellum Virginia*. Urbana: University of Illinois Press, 1978.

Saxon, A. H. P. T. *Barnum: The Legend and the Man*. New York: Columbia University Press, 1989.

Scott, M.D., James R., Philip J. DiSaia, M.D., Charles B. Hammond, M.D., and William N. Spellacy, M.D., eds. *Danforth's Obstetrics and Gynecology*. Sixth edition. Philadelphia: J. B. Lippincott, 1990.

Sedgwick, Eve Kosofsky. *Tendencies*. Durham: Duke University Press, 1993.

Shapiro, Michael. *The Politics of Representation: Writing Practices in Biography, Photography, and Policy Analysis*. Madison: University of Wisconsin Press, 1988.

Shapiro, Thomas M. *Population Control Politics: Women, Sterilization, and Reproductive Choice*. Philadelphia: Temple University Press, 1985.

Shaviro, Steven. *The Cinematic Body*. Minneapolis: University of Minnesota Press, 1993.

Shochet, M.D., Bernard R., Leon A. Levin, M.D., and Ephraim T. Lisansky, M.D. "Roundtable: The Seductive Patient." *Medical Aspects of Human Sexuality* 16, no. 1 (January 1982): 36F–36W.

Shohat, Ella. "'Laser for Ladies': Endo Discourse and the Inscriptions of Science." *Camera Obscura* 29 (May 1992): 57–90.

Showalter, Elaine. *The Female Malady: Women, Madness, and English Culture, 1830–1980*. New York: Viking Penguin, 1985.

Silverman, Kaja. "Masochism and Male Subjectivity." *Camera Obscura* 17 (1988): 30–67.

———. "Suture" (excerpts). In *Narrative, Apparatus, Ideology*. Edited by Philip Rosen. New York: Columbia University Press, 1988, pp. 219–35.

Sims, M.D., J. Marion. *The Story of My Life*. Edited by H. Marion-Sims, M.D. New York: D. Appleton and Company, 1886.

Smith, M.D., John M. *Women and Doctors*. New York: Atlantic Monthly Press, 1992.

Smith, Vicki L. "Sharing Ourselves . . . Our Greatest Strength." *Women Wise* 9, no. 2 (summer 1986): 6–7.

Solomon-Godeau, Abigail. *Photography at the Dock: Essays on Photographic History, Institutions, and Practices*. Minneapolis: University of Minnesota Press, 1990.

Speert, M.D., Harold. *Obstetric and Gynecologic Milestones*. New York: Macmillan, 1958.

Stabile, Carol A. "Shooting the Mother: Fetal Photography and the Politics of Disappearance." *Camera Obscura* 28 (1992): 178–205.

Stafford, Barbara Maria. *Body Criticism: Imaging the Unseen in Enlightenment Art and Medicine*. Cambridge: MIT Press, 1991.

Stalleybrass, Peter, and Allon White. *The Politics and Poetics of Transgression*. Ithaca: Cornell University Press, 1986.

Stewart, Susan. *On Longing: Narratives of the Miniature, the Gigantic, the Souvenir, the Collection*. Durham: Duke University Press, 1993.

Stone, Sandy. "The *Empire* Strikes Back: A Posttranssexual Manifesto." *Camera Obscura* 29 (1992): 151–78.

Straayer, Chris. "The Seduction of Boundaries: Feminist Fluidity in Annie Sprinkle's Art/Education/Sex." In *Dirty Looks: Women, Pornography, Power*. Edited by Pamela Church Gibson and Roma Gibson. London: British Film Institute, 1993, pp. 156–75.

Tanagho, M.D., Emile A., and Jack W. McAninch, M.D., eds. *Smith's General Urology*. 12th ed. Norwalk: Appleton and Lange, 1988.

Taussig, Michael. *Mimesis and Alterity: A Particular History of the Senses*. New York: Routledge, 1993.

Thorp, Jr. M.D., John M. "Patient Autonomy, Informed Consent, and Routine Episiotomy." *Contemporary OB/Gyn* 40, no. 9 (September 1995): 92–102

Treichler, Paula A., and Lisa Cartwright, eds. *Camera Obscura* 28–29 (1992).

Tyler, Stephen A. *The Unspeakable: Discourse, Dialogue, and Rhetoric in the Postmodern World*. Madison: University of Wisconsin Press, 1987.

Vaughan, M.D., Daniel G., ed. *General Ophthalmology*. 12th ed. Norwalk: Appleton and Lange, 1989.

Vontver, M.D., Louis, et al. "The Effects of Two Methods of Pelvic Examination Instruction on Student Performance and Anxiety." *Journal of Medical Education* 55 (September 1980): 778–85.

"Vulvar Self Exam." *Modern Medicine* 58 (February 1990): 30–31.

Wallis, M.D., Lilla A. "The Patient as Partner in the Pelvic Exam." *The Female Patient* 7 (March 1982): 28/4–28/7.

Wattleton, Faye. "Using Birth Control as Coercion." *Los Angeles Times*, January 13, 1991.

Weiss, Lawrence D. *No Benefit: Crisis in America's Health Insurance Industry*. Boulder: Westview, 1992.

Wertz, R. W., and D. W. Wertz. *Lying-in: A History of Childbirth in America*. New Haven: Yale University Press, 1977.

White, Deborah Gray. *Ar'n't I a Woman? Female Slaves in the Plantation South*. New York: W. W. Norton, 1985.

Williams, Linda. "A Provoking Agent: The Pornography and Performance Art of Annie Sprinkle." In *Dirty Looks*. Edited by Pamela Church Gibson and Roma Gibson. London: British Film Institute, 1993, pp. 176–91.

———. *Hard Core: Power, Pleasure, and the "Frenzy of the Visible."* Berkeley: University of California Press, 1989.

———. "Film Body: An Implantation of Perversions." In *Narrative, Apparatus, Ideology*. Edited by Philip Rosen. New York: Columbia University Press, 1988, pp. 507–34.

Wilson, Julie M. "The Pelvic Teaching Program at GWHC." *Sage-Femme* (winter 1978): 6.

Women's Community Health Center, Inc. "Experiences of a Pelvic Teaching Group." *Women and Health* 1 (July/August 1976): 19–23.

Wood, Ann Douglas. " 'The Fashionable Diseases': Women's Complaints and Their Treatment in Nineteenth-Century America." In *Women and Health in America*. Edited by Judith Walzer Leavitt. Madison: University of Wisconsin Press, 1984, pp. 222–38.

Wood, Robin. "Cronenberg: A Dissenting View." In *The Shape of Rage: The Films of David Cronenberg*. Edited by Piers Handling. New York: New York Zoetrope, 1983, pp. 115–35.

Word, M.D., S. Buford. "The Father of Gynecology." *Alabama Journal of Medical Science* 9, no. 1 (1972): 33–39.

Index

Terri Kapsalis is a health educator and performer. Her writings have appeared in
Lusitania, *New Formations*, *Public*, and *TDR*. She has taught in art schools and
medical schools and is currently teaching in the Department of Performance
Studies at Northwestern University.

Library of Congress Cataloging-in-Publication Data
Kapsalis, Terri.
Public privates : performing gynecology from both ends of the speculum / by Terri Kapsalis.
Includes bibliographical references and index.
ISBN 0-8223-1928-4 (alk. paper). — ISBN 0-8223-1921-7 (pbk. : alk. paper)
1. Gynecology—Social aspects.   2. Gynecology—Public opinion.   3. Gynecologists—
Attitudes.   4. Women patients—Public opinion.   I. Title.
RG103.K37   1997
618.1—dc20   96-29409 CIP